Here is what people are saying...

Andrea's philosophy of natural foods has opened my eyes to the many benefits of eating with care. I feel light and full of energy. *– Imma Giocoli*

If people knew that eating healthy would taste this good, I think everybody would be reformed. *– Linda Saul*

Andrea's recipes are delicious and very easy to cook – even for people who think they can't cook. Her food always makes me feel stronger, healthier and better after I eat it. *– Susan Weinstein*

By adding wholesome organic products into my diet I have been able to eliminate refined sugar intake on a daily basis. I also have Graves disease, a hyperthyroid condition, and have been able to stay in remission by balancing my life and food. *– Karyn Bender*

What a great combination; great food, easy recipes and comedy all together. The laughter is the perfect seasoning for all the delicious foods. *– Mary Lou Minard*

I was afraid that I would have to spend hours in the kitchen if I cooked whole foods. Surprisingly, it takes about the same time to prepare a healthy meal as it does to order take-out! *– Jason Poole*

Andrea's cooking manages to be both healthful and tasty. I love that she takes simple, natural ingredients and turns them into masterpieces. *– Teresa Theophano*

I feel better, I'm cooking more now, and I feel more at peace. *– Amy Botelho*

Andrea is an inspiration – she has made me aware that abundant health is attainable; she is living proof of that. *– Margaret Vuletic*

Andrea has taught me that it is so important to understand and implement a deeper level of awareness when it comes to food, nourishment and healing. I have certainly been able to feel a huge difference in my body. *– Laura Hames*

BETTER FOOD, BETTER HEALTH

THE
Whole
Truth

Eating & Recipe Guide

Andrea Beaman
HHC, AADP

This book is not intended as a substitute for medical advice from a physician.
The material contained in *The Whole Truth Eating & Recipe Guide*, is for general
information and the purpose of educating individuals on nutrition, lifestyle,
health & fitness and related topics. Should you have any health care related
questions, please consult with your physician or other qualified health care
provider before embarking on a new treatment, diet, fitness or exercise program.

Cover design Julie Mueller
jam graphics & design

TABLE OF CONTENTS

PART I
BETTER FOOD

PART II
BETTER FOOD RECIPES

GREAT GRAINS

BOUNTIFUL BEANS

DELICIOUS DESSERTS

ACKNOWLEDGEMENTS

I believe, with a solid support system, anything is possible - and I have been blessed with one. First and foremost, I want to thank my father, Richard Beaman, for being my biggest fan and the greatest role model. I love you, Dad – you are my hero.

Thank you Erica for the fantastic editing job and content suggestions; you are the best sister and friend I could ever ask for. And, thank you to the rest of my family for love, reinforcement and encouragement: Marc & Donna, Marc Anthony, Andrew, Brandon, Ricky & Imma, Terry, Uncle Al, Lyndon, Danny and the newest addition to the family, Phil. A strong family foundation is invaluable to my continued success.

Thank you to my amazing community of friends and peers who inspire me to be the best I can be: Katharine McMaster, Kim Gantz-Wexler, Dina & Dave Marro (yes, Dave… just your mere existence in the world, and the love you share with my friend is vital to my creativity!), Jeannie & Anthony DelGreco – thank you for growing with me, Robert Parker, Linda Nealon, Julie Austin, Delia Quigley, Joshua Rosenthal and The Institute For Integrative Nutrition. This is truly a roll call of greatness, and I am blessed to know you all.

Thank you to my clients and cooking class students for letting me test these delicious recipes on your beautiful, willing taste buds! And, a great big thanks to all of the chefs and restaurateurs who support organic foods, sustainable agriculture, and purchase from local farms to ensure the best food gets served while preserving the integrity of the planet: Joy & Bart at Candle Café and Candle 79, Tom Colicchio of Gramercy Tavern and Craft, Alice Waters of Chez Panisse, Louis Lanza of Josie's and Better Burger, Dan Barber of Blue Hill, and countless others who consistently and consciously feed people great quality food.

And, last but certainly not least, thank you to all the farmers around the world who tend to the food supply without using toxic chemicals and pesticides – you are keeping the food clean and safe for human consumption. Thank you for feeding me!

INTRODUCTION

My experience with food while growing up was *not* a healthy one. I mindlessly ate food with no concept of its effect on my body or long-term health. By the time I was a teenager my daily diet consisted of everything fat-free, low-fat, sugar-free, diet and lo-cal, and yet I couldn't seem to escape the chronic dieting syndrome that kept me climbing up and down on that darn bathroom scale! I was trapped in a dieting mindset and food had become my enemy.

There are an overwhelming number of diet plans on the market and I experimented with most of them, but still had no idea that reaching my ideal weight was first and foremost a result of overall bodily *health*. To permanently live at or near your ideal weight the body must enter into—and remain in—a state of health. And, my *health* is what I neglected while I focused on weight loss.

The highly processed, chemical-laden *non* food substances I was consuming on a daily basis contained virtually no nutrients. And, although I was "chunky," my body was literally starving for vitamins and minerals and began to physically break down; I was exhausted, chronically sick with flu and colds, had a weak immune system, and needed constant stimulation from coffee and sugary sweets to acquire energy.

It was not until my mother's second diagnosis of breast cancer that I began to wonder about the direct effect food had on health. As I supported my mother and walked along side her throughout her illness, I slowly educated myself about *real* food. By the time my mother passed away, the connection between better food and better health was clear, but I was young and ignorant and didn't utilize the information to prevent future illnesses from manifesting in my own body.

I continued eating poor quality non food substances (diet soda, artificial sweeteners, diet foods, highly refined foods, etc.) and over time my eating habits had created within me an unhealthy environment enabling a debilitating disease to take root and grow. In my late twenties, I was diagnosed with thyroid disease and informed there was "no cure." The doctors advised me I would need to take a prescription medication for the rest of my life.

Thankfully, a lifetime of medication with "no cure" was not on my agenda. Instead, I simply applied the information I learned about food when my mother was sick. I knew the food I was eating on a daily basis directly paralleled my relationship to sickness, and would ultimately parallel my relationship to health. Weight loss was no longer a factor in my life – *true health* was my new goal.

My life monumentally transformed once I changed my mind about "dieting" and incorporated real food that was wholesome, organic, nutritious, tasty, and seasonal. I know today that maintaining a tight focus on *weight loss* is a self-defeating plan of action: as long as the body is unhealthy, weight can never be properly maintained. The only lasting approach to weight loss is a holistic one, a method that aims to achieve the health of the total being.

Utilizing food as a health-promoting tool allowed me to make food a great tasting ally instead of the enemy I once believed it was. *This Whole Truth Eating and Recipe Guide* is designed to help you discover the best quality foods to promote better health and how to make them taste absolutely delicious.

4

Contrary to what some people may think, healthier food does not have to be boring, bland, difficult to prepare, or expensive. Taste is a HUGE factor for me, as it is for many people. If it doesn't taste good, I don't care how healthy it is, I'm not going to eat it and neither should you. You will soon realize that eating better quality food is not only pleasurable, but can improve your health at the same time.

I no longer carelessly throw food into my body; I have a nourishing relationship with the food I eat. Eating has become a fully immersed, enjoyable experience where I properly fuel myself with the most fantastic tasting foods that are appropriate for me. Food can, and should, be a wonderful experience that enhances your life – I know it did mine, and many clients too.

Better health didn't happen overnight, it was an on-going process that became more evident as I deepened my awareness and understanding of food, and began to eat in a more natural way. Within four months I lost about twenty pounds, and within two years I naturally healed my thyroid disease without medication. That was almost a decade ago, and I've never had to "diet" again. Achieving my ideal weight happened effortlessly as my health improved.

Eating "healthfully" isn't about deprivation or dieting; it's about changing the *quality* of food to reap the benefits from it. It's about making your food work for you to nourish your body, instead of working against you, depleting vitality. It's about wholly satisfying your body with delicious, nutritious meals and not starving yourself to death, or creating deficiencies while on fad diets!

As you read through this Eating and Recipe Guide, I'll explain *why* we eat specific foods at certain times of the year, describe each of those foods in detail (energetically and scientifically), and then offer simple, scrumptious recipes for you to experiment with in your kitchen and in your body.

Keep in mind, there is not one specific diet for all people. Everyone is unique and we all have different physical, environmental, and nutritional needs. This guide can help you better understand your bodily needs, and with that knowledge you can create exactly the kind of meals to help you reach your health-related goals, whatever they may be.

It will take some persistence and patience at first as you learn how and why to incorporate new foods. But, the more you show up at the "plate" and make better food choices as often as possible, the more opportunity you'll have to hit a home run for your health!

Hippocrates, the father of medicine said, "Let food be thy medicine, and medicine be thy food." I believe food is medicinal and can help you look and feel your absolute best, meal after delicious meal.

Now…it's time to learn about food and then get into the kitchen and cook up some yummy dishes for you and your family, friends and loved ones.

Eat well, live long, and enjoy every mouthwatering meal.

Better food for better health,
Andrea Beaman, HHC, AADP
Holistic Health Counselor
American Association of Drugless Practitioners

Part I

BETTER FOODS

CHAPTER 1

FOOD GLORIOUS FOOD

I *hated* food when I was growing up. I bet you didn't expect an opening sentence like that in a chapter entitled Food Glorious Food! But, it's true... I hated food because I didn't understand it or its effect on me. How could I eat fat-free, non-fat, low-fat, sugar-free, diet foods and yet never seem to reach a satisfying weight or feel comfortable in my body? It was confusing and frustrating. I attempted to starve myself into thinness by taking (and getting addicted to) prescription diet pills and over the counter diet pills. I wouldn't eat for days at a time. Yet, I still I couldn't achieve my ideal weight. I would lose weight for brief periods, but would always gain it back, plus some. Eventually, food became my sworn enemy and for many years I wanted it out of my body in any way I could get it out; bingeing and purging, and laxatives helped. Unfortunately, I *had* to continue eating for survival so I kept returning for more food even though I found no joy in it. My relationship with food was highly dysfunctional and I needed serious food therapy. I finally got it, in the form of a disease.

Throughout my teenage and young adult years I was chronically sick with flu and colds, herpes simplex I, allergies, acne, digestive problems, yo-yo weight issues and then finally in my late-twenties I was diagnosed with thyroid disease. It was a *blessing*. I needed that disease to shake some sense into me.

As recounted in my first book The Whole Truth - How I Naturally Reclaimed My Health and You Can Too, I witnessed my mother's unsuccessful battle with breast cancer using modern medicine as the doctors recommended. After my diagnosis with thyroid disease, I had no desire to lay down my arms and surrender to the prescribed medical route suggested to me. A lifetime of medication with no cure was not on my agenda. Instead, I altered my dysfunctional diet and lifestyle and healed myself naturally.

My physical condition dramatically recovered when I learned how to make food a great tasting ally instead of the enemy I believed it was. Today, I *love, love, love* food. I couldn't imagine a day without it. And, I love to feel good about the food I eat and know its effect on my body and mind. My relationship with food has changed, but I could have never achieved that level of gratification while stuck on a "diet" focusing solely on weight loss.

There are so many diets out on the market that attempting to figure out what type of food to eat can be overwhelming to say the least. I tried the grapefruit diet, the cabbage soup diet (that one was a real gas!), the meal replacement diet, the liquid diet, the fat-free diet, the high protein diet, Weight Watchers, Jenny Craig, The Vegan Diet, and countless others. Many of them had good information, but all were lacking in one thing or another, which ultimately kept *me* lacking in one thing or another… mainly my health. I finally reached my ideal weight when I stopped dieting altogether and began making the best possible food choices for the sake of my health instead.

Calorie restricting diets or adhering to strict food plans, don't work in the long term – they never have and they never will. Diets are not designed to create lasting health, they are designed primarily for weight loss, and that can come at a huge cost. First and foremost, to your sanity! As long as you are "dieting" you could be trapped in a state of deprivation that can lead to bouts of obsessive calorie counting, fat cutting, weighing of food portions, restricting carbohydrate, starvation rituals, and an overall lack of pleasure around eating food.

The information contained within these pages is *not* about creating another fad diet. This Eating and Recipe guide is designed to teach you how to make the best food choices to help you achieve vibrant health, and with that, your ideal weight can be reached effortlessly. Eating better quality food will keep you out of the calorie-counting cuckoo's nest and fully enjoying food.

Knowing what to eat should be a simple and pleasurable experience, but for many of us food choices can create panic instead – and for good reasons. In the last century *food experts* have told us to fear fat, so everyone switched to fat-free foods and butter substitutes like margarine. Now they're telling us margarine is worse for your health than butter. Then they told us to fear sugar and everything became sugar free and the artificial sweetener industry boomed. Today, the links between disease and artificial sweeteners is growing.[1] Then they told us to fear red meat, and vegetarianism and veganism exploded onto the marketplace – faux meats made from soy and other substances became fashionable. Then they told us to fear carbohydrates and carbophobia was borne – bread makers around the world, with their fiery ovens, were thought to be doing the devil's work! Currently, scientists are dissecting each particular food to discover its individual healthful properties (antioxidants and

---

[1] http://www.sweetpoison.com/

phytonutrients), which has *some* validity, but as a whole completely misses the mark (which you'll soon discover as you continue reading). There is so much conflicting information about food it's no wonder people are paralyzed and stuck in the dieting industry. Where there is a lack of knowledge there is fear.

As you increase your knowledge about food, you will gain the power to fearlessly make the best possible choices for your health. By making *real* food choices, you'll realize that you will never need to diet again.

I know you may be thinking that you already are eating *real* food, but if you are plagued with illness, exhaustion, an overweight condition, achy bones and joints, or sick and suffering in any way, chances are you are not eating real food, or you are eating food that might not be appropriate for you.

Much of what we're eating today is highly refined and chemicalized substances that merely resemble food, but are not nourishing to our body or mind. Any food that is processed, packaged, preserved with chemicals, enhanced with artificial sweeteners, or labeled fat-free, low-fat, skim, carb-free, diet, or sugar-free, can fall into this "non-food" category. These particular foods lack many of the essential nutrients needed to create vitality and will require us to eat more and more of them to feel satisfied. Eating these non-foods on a regular basis leaves us physically deficient and unable to reach the level of fulfillment that comes with eating wholesome meals. A good rule of thumb to remember, if the word "free" is somewhere on the package, chances are you may be paying the price with your health.

If the food you are eating is nutritionally deficient, unsatisfying or inappropriate, the need to overeat remains as your body searches for the proper amount of fuel it needs to thrive. Eating non-food substances leaves us overweight and unhealthy, and prone to dieting to help us lose the weight. It's a vicious cycle. The best way to break this pattern is to improve your understanding of food, change the quality of your food, and then begin eating whole foods that are nourishing and delicious.

Read the insights about better food sources and begin incorporating the philosophies contained herein, and you'll be able to achieve your health related goals no matter what they are. This guide is about making smarter food choices to enhance your overall health. There are no charts detailing specific quantities of protein, fat, carbohydrate, or portion sizes. Everyone is unique and each body has its own set of nutritional requirements. A construction worker wielding heavy tools all day will need more fuel (food) in his system than a librarian sitting at a desk. It's common sense that one diet does not fit everyone's needs. The information in this guide is designed to help raise your consciousness about food so you can ultimately figure out what is best for you as an individual.

Deepening your knowledge of food will guide you toward creating a healthier relationship to what you're eating. If you were dating and seeking an appropriate partner you would actively pursue someone who is good for you. Right? I want you to create a similar aspiration with food – choose food that is good for you. And of course, choose foods that are mouthwatering and delicious! Essentially, it's time for you to have a nourishing love affair with the foods you take into your beautiful body.

The following chapters explain food sources and their potential effects. It's up to you to decide what to do with the information. If you are plagued with illness, weight problems or are just seeking better health, I suggest you incorporate some of the ideas, and easy recipes into your life. You have nothing to lose (except excess weight and potential illness!), and everything to gain – like better health.

TASTY TIDBITS

- Identify all non-food items in your home (highly refined packaged foods, sugar-free, fat-free, butter substitutes, diet food, fake meats, artificial sweeteners, etc.) and toss into the garbage. Okay, you can have one last bite, but that's it!
- Think about all the diets you've tried in the past and list them on a piece of paper. Crumple up the paper and throw it into the garbage.
- Take out the garbage.
- Change your focus from losing weight to improving health.
- Open your mind to learning about better food choices.
- There's nothing to fear.

CHAPTER 2
GREAT GRAINS

For thousands of years whole grains have been a traditional food for much of the world's populations. Europeans ate buckwheat, barley and rye, Asians dined on millet and rice, Africans consumed teff, South Americans feasted on quinoa and amaranth, and in North America we munched on maize and wheat – to name a few.

Whole grains are comprised of some of the major nutrients the body needs to thrive; vitamins, minerals, fat, protein, carbohydrates, and fiber. According to many studies, including one at the University of Minnesota, "A diet rich in whole grains lowers body mass index, lowers total cholesterol, and lowers waist-to-hip ratios. Various large epidemiological studies on a variety of different populations note that people who eat three daily servings of whole grains have been shown to reduce their risk of heart disease by 25-36%, stroke by 37%, Type II diabetes by 21-27%, digestive system cancers by 21-43%, and hormone-related cancers by 10-40%. Furthermore, in intervention studies where whole grains became a regular part of the diet, people showed improved blood glucose levels and insulin sensitivity."[2]

Our ancestors didn't have access to any of the above scientific data we know today, but somehow they must have intuitively known there

---

[2] http://www.wholegrain.umn.edu/health/index.cfm

were benefits to eating wholesome, nutrient rich grains; otherwise they wouldn't have eaten them.

We are still eating grains today but unfortunately, most are highly refined, simple carbohydrates (cakes, pastries, cookies, processed cereals, white rice, white flour products, etc.). The difference between whole grains and refined grains is vast: whole grains are a complete food with its beneficial nutrients intact, while refined grains have lost most of these vital elements during the milling process. As disease rates skyrocket in modern society, it's becoming evident that the extreme refining of grains has left us as physically deficient as the foods we're consuming.

In addition to losing nutritional value, the starches in highly refined grains are absorbed *quickly*, upsetting blood sugar levels that the body regulates by releasing insulin. Persistent blood sugar instability can eventually lead to debilitating ailments like diabetes (and all of its complications), and heart disease.[3] On the other hand, the natural and complex sugars in whole grains are broken down *slowly* into glucose molecules that enter the small intestine and supply the body with steady sustainable energy. Cognitive power, among other bodily functions, requires glucose. That means whole grains are especially nourishing for the brain.

Energetically, whole grains have been used to calm the mind, contribute to a good night's sleep, create balance, satisfy hunger, promote smooth bowel movements, long memory, and clear thinking.[4] Ponder this... whole grains retain the integrity (wholeness) to create whole thoughts. Now that really is "food for thought!"

---

[3] http://scc.healthcentral.com/bcp/main.asp?page=newsdetail&id=521255&ap=93&brand=24
[4] Healing with Whole Foods, by Paul Pitchford, North Atlantic Books, 1993, pg.416

Whole grains were traditionally prepared by soaking, sprouting (germinating the seed) or fermenting, which rendered them more digestible, and increased nutritional potency. Today, by rushing to produce food for the mass market, many of those essential preparation techniques have been skipped. This may be one of the reasons why highly refined wheat flour and other cereal grains can cause allergies or other negative reactions in some people.

According to traditional foods chef and author, Sally Fallon, "All grains contain phytic acid in the outer layer or bran. Untreated phytic acid can combine with calcium, magnesium, copper, iron and especially zinc, in the intestinal tract and block their absorption."[5]

Refining the grain by stripping the outer bran eliminates the phytic acid, but also eliminates essential nutrients, bran and fiber. Eating a diet of improperly prepared (untreated) and refined grains can have a weakening effect on the body instead of a strengthening one, so it's best to use traditional methods and thank our ancestors for their wise knowledge. Soaking grains is not as long a process as one may think. All that is required is some advance planning. It's as easy as putting grains in a bowl, covering with water and setting on the kitchen counter before going to bed, or before leaving for work in the morning. Voila! Done! Grains can soak for eight to twenty-four hours, and some cultures soak grains for up to three days, so you don't have to worry about over-soaking. When you're ready to prepare the grains, discard the soaking water and cook with fresh water according to the recipe. Grains like brown rice, millet, kasha and quinoa have lower levels of phytic acid and don't necessarily need to be soaked.

---

[5] *Nourishing Traditions*, by Sally Fallon, New Trends Publishing, 2001, p452

The heartier grains like wheat and rye can be difficult to digest in their whole unprocessed form and were customarily prepared by soaking, sprouting, and then grinding into flour, or fermenting to form naturally leavened breads (like sourdough). Properly prepared whole grain breads, although partially refined, are not less wholesome but are easier to digest, increasing their nutritional benefit. Sprouted grain breads, sourdough breads, and other whole grain products can be purchased in any health food store, gourmet market and most supermarkets too. Some places you'll most likely find these products are at any Whole Foods Market, Trader Joes, Wild Oats, Wild By Nature, or any local health food store. There is a **Resources** page in the back of this guide to help you locate whatever you need.

Read the label on whole grain breads or other products to make sure you can pronounce everything on the ingredient list. If you stumble across words you couldn't spell with your eyes closed, it's a sure sign that it may not be a "real" food. Generally speaking… the more simple the ingredients the more wholesome the food.

Another way to properly "treat" grains is by chewing them. The simple act of chewing food may have never been taught to some, or has been forgotten by most people, including myself! When I was growing up my mother and father would tell me to "chew your food." But, I didn't listen to the wise advice from my parents (who does?). Instead, eating was more of a shoveling and swallowing experience for me. The only thing I consciously chewed was big wads of bubble-gum!

Chewing releases a carbohydrate-digesting enzyme, ptyalin, which increases absorption of nutrients and aids digestion. And, chewing consciously slows down the eating process, giving the body and mind the

18

opportunity to recognize that it might not need as much food as may be piled on the plate. Gandhi said, "Drink your food and chew your drink." Smart guy. If I had listened to Gandhi and my parents with regard to chewing (as well as many other things!), I might have had better health.

It's time to use your beautiful teeth for more than just smiling in pictures, so chew, chew, chew your food. However, continue to smile as often as possible because laughter is great medicine. But, please make sure you finish chewing first! Especially, if you're chewing something green that has a tendency to lodge directly between your two front teeth.

Various whole grains to chew include barley, brown rice, rye, wheat, corn, millet, buckwheat (kasha), quinoa, amaranth, teff, oats, wild rice, maize, spelt, and kamut. Each grain has its own unique energy. Begin experimenting with one of the most common grains, brown rice, and eat it daily for an entire week to observe your body's reaction. Within a short amount of time you may notice bowel movements have become more regular and sleep patterns may change too.

My body physically changed, and many of my clients' too. Prior to improving my diet I was often constipated, and would also wake two or three times per night to urinate. These were subtle signals of failing health, but I didn't make the connection. After incorporating whole grains and other natural foods into my diet those dysfunctions became a distant memory of my unhealthy past.

Eating whole grains doesn't mean that refined grains are completely nixed off the menu. It can be healthy and fun to eat lightly refined grains like cous-cous, bulghur, pasta, and breads, and other highly refined grain products including cookies, cakes and pastries, too! The key to achieving better health is to eat whole grains and whole grain products *most* often and highly refined grains *least* often.

I do not keep white bread, white rice or white sugar in my home but, when I dine at a restaurant or a friend's house, I may not have access to a better choice. I always ask if they have whole grain bread or brown rice and most do. If a better option is not available I let myself enjoy what the environment provides knowing that one piece of white bread isn't going to destroy my health. It's not what I do once in a while that harms my body it's what I do on a daily basis.

The scientific facts and figures about eating whole grains are out there, and it's time to put them to good use, inside your body, where they can benefit you most. The whole truth about whole foods and real nutrition is essential to helping you realize your long-term health goals.

If you're getting hungry with all this talk of food, skip to the recipe section and cook the Sauteed Shrimp with Vegetables and Plum Sauce and lay it on top of long grain brown rice. Chew, chew, chew it well. Then come on back and continue reading about better quality foods!

TASTY TIDBITS

- Identify the highly refined grain products in your home (donuts, pastries, cookies, cakes, pretzels, snack foods, white bread, white rice) and toss into the garbage or feed it to the birds (try not to kill them!).

- Replace white rice with brown rice, and white bread with whole grain bread.

- Chew your food at least twenty-five times or until it turns to liquid in your mouth.

- Make better food choices as often as possible.

- The Resources list in the back of this guide will help you locate stores in your area, organic foods, and any other products you need.

- When eating away from home remember to *ask* if there is a whole grain option.

- Listen to the wise advice of your parents, sages and ancestors (and me, of course).

CHAPTER 3

VERITABLE VEGETABLE HARVEST

Vegetables contain a wide spectrum of vitamins, minerals, phytonutrients and antioxidants: vitamin A, beta carotene, lycopene, sulphoraphane, vitamins B1, B2, B5, B6, niacin, folacin, vitamin C, vitamin E, vitamin K, coenzyme Q10, boron, calcium, silicon, germanium, iron, magnesium, manganese, potassium, selenium, sulfur, zinc, amino acids, enzymes, and more. The list of nutritional benefits within this category of food is long and delicious!

Unfortunately, the scientific information regarding the importance of vitamins and minerals has been exploited, and thus, the supplement industry was borne. Within the past few decades, masses of people seeking health run out to buy supplements believing isolated nutrients will magically enhance health, but it doesn't. Vitamin and mineral supplements are partial foods, and long-term use can have detrimental effects, outweighing the initial good they may do.

Like many people, I used to spend hundreds of dollars (and more) on supplements, ingesting ten to fifteen per day seeking a quick fix. The short-term effects and slight boost in energy initially made me feel better, but still I became quite ill with thyroid disease and overall poor health.

Ingesting excessive amounts of highly refined vitamins and minerals, combined with long term use, can contribute to many physical dysfunctions including:

- Vitamin A - liver damage and birth defects
- Folic acid - increased risk of neurological disorders
- Vitamin B6 - nerve damage
- Vitamin C - anemia, calcification of the arteries and kidney stones
- Vitamin E - excessive bleeding[6]

Supplementing is *not* the best way to achieve lasting health. Using real foods to acquire vitamins and minerals is a better option, without the negative side effects. A carrot for example not only contains beta carotene but, a host of other vitamins, minerals, water, carbohydrate, fiber, and natural sugars. The body requires *all* of the carrot's properties to properly digest and absorb its nutrients. And, the physical process of *eating* a carrot satisfies the senses as well as creates a well-rounded gastronomical experience.

Try this experiment: drizzle extra virgin olive oil on a bunch of fresh carrots. Add minced rosemary, a pinch of sea salt, and bake at 375° for forty-five minutes or until soft and sweet. Place the carrots on a dinner plate and set it on the table. Then take a small round, hard, gelatin coated beta-carotene supplement, place that on a dinner plate and set it on the table next to the roasted carrots. You can clearly see, smell, and taste the difference. Opting for a pill instead of eating tasty food can deprive the body and mind from a delicious eating experience. Great health and physical fulfillment can be better achieved by *eating* the source of the vitamins and minerals.

Generally speaking, there are three categories of vegetables to choose from (of course there are more than three, but let's not make this

---

[6] All About Vitamin Pills", Newsweek, January 20, 2003, p. 51

complicated!). There are leafy greens, ground or round, and root
vegetables.

Leafy green vegetables include arugula, broccoli rappini, bok
choy, chinese cabbage, chives, cilantro, collard greens, dandelion greens,
endive, escarole, kale, leeks, lettuces, mustard greens, parsley, scallions,
spinach, swiss chard, watercress and others. These vegetables are rich in
chlorophyll, can purify and oxygenate the blood, deodorize bad breath and
body odor (nice bonus!), improve liver function, help to reduce high blood
pressure and much more.

Energetically, leafy greens grow up out of the ground, toward the
sky. Eating these vegetables can lighten us up, lift the spirits, and impart
into us that same "upward" energy. If you're feeling down, leafy greens
can be better than taking anti-depressants!

When I first tried dark leafy green vegetables I didn't appreciate
their strong bitter flavor. I met a natural foods counselor who told me
there would come a time when I would crave kale. Imagine that? Of all
the things to crave… kale! Egads, I laughed and told him he was crazy.
He was the one to have the last laugh though. Two months after
improving my diet I actually craved kale and ate it three times a day:
breakfast, lunch and dinner. I was a leafy green eatin' machine. I listened
to my body, gave it what it craved, and every day I grew healthier.
Eventually, my body fueled up with the proper amount of nutrition it
needed and my kale cravings naturally reduced. I still love kale, but I
don't eat it three times per day.

Our second group of vegetables is the round and ground category.
They grow at the surface on the ground (or directly underneath it) and
include acorn squash, broccoli, butternut squash, green and red cabbage,

cauliflower, celeriac, cucumber, delicata squash, garlic, green beans, green peas, potatoes, hokkaido pumpkin, hubbard squash, mushrooms, onions, patty pan squash, pumpkin, radishes, summer squash, zucchini and many others.

Energetically, these vegetables nourish the center (mid-section) of the body and can have a centering and balancing effect. Sweet vegetables like onions, squash and cabbage help to relax the body and can curb incessant sweet cravings too.

A young male client in his mid-thirties was complaining about his insatiable sweet tooth and uncomfortable tight muscle condition. I recommended he incorporate sweet vegetables like onion, cabbage and winter squash into his diet. A few weeks later he returned for a follow-up visit and seemed much more relaxed. He told me his muscles felt less constricted and his massage therapist noticed the change also. And, although he was still craving sweets, it was much less. His one-box-per-sitting graham cracker habit had been reduced to one sleeve (four sleeves in a box). That's what I call progress!

Now, it's time to dig down deep into the earth and discover the benefits of the third category of vegetables - roots. This includes: beets, ginger, carrots, parsnips, burdock, daikon, parsley root, rutabaga, turnips, and others.

Root vegetables grow down into the ground and have a strong descending energy aiding physical and emotional stability. Root vegetables do exactly what the name implies: they can make you feel rooted. I suggest eating hearty roots to acquire the steadfast energy needed to take on the task of healing your beautiful body. So... grab a shovel and dig in!

26

Our vegetable section wouldn't be complete without the addition of culinary herbs. For centuries herbs have been used as flavor enhancers and digestive aids. Including fresh and dried herbs into your meals is a wise and tasty choice. Below is information about some common herbs and their traditional medicinal benefits.

- **Basil** - natural diuretic, calms the nervous system, and stimulates appetite. Basil has a sweet flavor and blends well with most anything, even fruits (especially tomatoes).
- **Chives** – member of the allium family (onion), spicy, pungent flavor, rich in vitamin C, calcium, phosphorous, iron and enzymes. Chives go great with potatoes, butter, dips and spreads.
- **Cilantro** - soothes the stomach and intestines. Add this herb at the *end* of cooking to help retain its aromatic and distinct flavor. Cilantro tastes great in salsas, beans, salads and more.
- **Dill** - cooling energy, used to strengthen the stomach, and treat indigestion. Traditionally, dill has been used in pickles and pickled foods (grape leaves), salad dressing and fish dishes.
- **Fennel** - treats bad breath, alleviates gas (whew!), nausea and gout. Used in Mediterranean and Asian cooking, but you can use it in any type of food.
- **Marjoram** - promotes digestion and stimulates the appetite. This herb is similar in flavor to oregano only milder. Can be used in many meat dishes, or any recipe that calls for oregano.
- **Mint** - eases indigestion, fatigue, headache and fever. Its natural menthol flavor is good for clearing congestion. Mint is excellent in salads and desserts.

- **Oregano** - is a natural decongestant, anti-inflammatory and antibacterial. Oregano is associated with Italian flavored dishes, but can be used in almost any recipe if you'd like.
- **Parsley** - contains high levels of calcium, chlorophyll, vitamins A, C, E and iron, and is a natural breath freshener (sweet bonus!). Parsley is great for flavoring stews, sauces and stocks, and to add a little zing of freshness to the plate.
- **Rosemary** - rich in antioxidants and used medicinally to promote circulation and calm the nervous system. Great flavor enhancer for roasted foods and hearty stews.
- **Sage** - counteracts intestinal inflammation and improves digestion of fat (maybe that's why it's traditionally used in so many holiday stuffing recipes!).
- **Tarragon** - natural diuretic and digestive stimulant. This herb blends well with meat dishes and sauces.
- **Thyme** - aids digestion, natural decongestant, treats diarrhea, hangovers and menstrual cramps. Traditionally used in herbs de Provence, meat dishes and sauces.[7]

There are many other herbs to choose from that enhance the flavor and healing ability of food. If fresh herbs are not available, dried herbs can be substituted.

Entire books have been written about the *scientific* benefits of antioxidant, vitamin and mineral rich vegetables, but I want to keep it

---

[7] Green Cuisine by Elisa Bosley, Delicious Living Magazine, pp.63-65

simple and not overload your mind with too many facts and figures to digest (pun intended here). All you really need to know is that vegetables can be an excellent addition to your daily diet, but to obtain great health all we really need to do is make them taste delicious and eat them!

TASTY TIDBITS

- Begin investing your money on *real* sources of vitamins and minerals, and when you're ready… toss those expensive supplements into the garbage.
- Incorporate a new vegetable into your diet every week.
- Try something from each category: leafy greens, ground, and root vegetables.
- Use fresh or dried herbs in your cooking to enhance flavor and improve digestion.
- Remember what your grandmother and mother used to say, "Shush up, and eat your veggies!"

CHAPTER 4

BOUNTIFUL BEANS AND LEGUMES

When I was growing up, my siblings and I would chant a popular little ditty that sounded something like this… "Beans, beans, they're good for your heart, the more you eat em', the more you ..." uhm... well let's just say they're good for the heart and the rest of your body too!

Beans are rich in plant protein, carbohydrates, unsaturated fats, vitamins, minerals, antioxidants, fiber and enzymes. Beans help regulate glucose metabolism, produce a slow rise in blood sugar, provide calm energy, and reduce the risk for heart disease and certain cancers.[8] [9] [10]

"Men with high cholesterol who ate a diet including a half cup daily of dried pinto, navy, kidney, and other beans had an average drop in cholesterol levels of 20 percent after three weeks."[11]

All that healthy information is good to know, but even better… beans actually taste good. Humans from all over the world have been consuming beans for centuries, "The cultivation of kidney beans in Central America goes back as far as 5000 BC, and pea seeds have been

---

[8] http://www.beansforhealth.org/

[9] http://www.truestarhealth.com/Notes/2015000.html

[10] http://www.whfoods.com/genpage.php?tname=foodspice&dbid=2

[11] J.W. Anderson and W.L. Chen, "Effect of Legumes and Their Soluble Fibers on Cholesterol-Rich Lipoproteins," American Chemical Society Abstracts AGFD #39, 1982. "Let Food Be Thy Medicine," by Alex Jack, One Peaceful World, 1999, p. 35.

found in the tombs of pharaohs who thought them to be good food for the afterworld."[12]

Beans and grains naturally compliment each other and have traditionally been served together to enhance nutritional value: rice and beans, hummus (chickpeas) and pita bread, dahl (lentils) and nan bread, black beans and corn (tortillas), pasta fagiole (bean and pasta soup), and others. Check out the Black Bean Burritos recipe in Part II – Better Food Recipes.

Beans are a delicious addition to a healthy diet, but can get a bad rap because some people have difficulty digesting them (hence the popularity of that childhood chant). First and foremost, the digestive system in many people is severely compromised from eating too many refined grains, sugars, and the overuse of antibiotics that contributes to the destruction of good intestinal bacteria, inhibiting digestion. Additional information on good and bad bacteria will be covered in greater detail in the chapter, Pickle-icious Foods.

Secondly, beans need to be properly prepared. This includes soaking them for eight to twenty-four hours to release acids, gas-causing enzymes and trisaccharides. Soaking beans with a small piece of kombu or kelp (sea vegetable), or adding one tablespoon of vinegar, softens the tough fibers, rendering them more digestible and producing less gas.

I'm not going to kid you here, beans do take time to prepare, but they are worth it. Smaller beans like lentils and adukis can be cooked within one hour, but larger beans like kidney, garbanzo, and cannelini can take two hours or longer. For some people spending two hours in the kitchen can seem like a life sentence! I know we're all busy, so if you do

---

[12] The Energetics Of Food, Steve Gagne, Spiral Sciences 1990, p232

not have the desire or time to prepare beans from scratch there are a variety of pre-cooked canned beans to choose from that can be purchased at your local health food store or supermarket.

If you can carve out the time on a Saturday or Sunday afternoon, put a large pot of beans on the stove while you clean up the house or do the laundry and within a couple of hours you could have prepared beans for the week. Cooking in bulk is a great way to save time when you are busy during the work week and can't find the time to cook. You could store the cooked beans in a sealed container and use it when needed. With beans already prepared you could easily throw together hearty bean stews, bean burritos, bean dips, rice and bean dishes and much more. *Timesaving Tips, Meals In Minutes and other Lifestyle Strategies* can be found in "The Whole Truth Ultimate Survival Guide."

Beans are members of the Leguminosae family or pulses, and include lentils, kidney, garbanzo, black beans, navy, northern, cannelini, pinto, lima, red, anasazi (red and white colored bean), black-eyed peas, green peas, split peas, and soybeans.

Traditionally fermented soybean products have been a healthy staple in many Asian cultures. These products include tofu, tempeh, miso, shoyu, natto and tamari. Keep in mind that these foods were generally eaten in small quantities. Sometimes people seeking health overeat something because it has been scientifically proven to have healing benefits, but always remember that "quantity, changes quality." The recipes in this book will guide you toward understanding "healthy" amounts.

A note of caution regarding improperly processed soy products. In America we've mass produced the soybean, exploited it, and it has now become an unhealthy food. Soybeans that aren't properly processed through traditional sprouting and fermenting methods have been linked with thyroid disease, digestive problems, reproductive disorders, cancer and other illnesses.[13]

Some "not-so-healthy" soy products include: isolated soy proteins, soy dogs, soy burgers, soy meats, soymilk, soy bars, soy ice cream, soybean oil, soy yogurts, soy margarine, soy nuts, and much more. If it's not *traditionally* made, odds are it's not good for your health despite it's popularity. Highly processed soy foods are "health-food junk foods" so don't eat large quantities (if any at all).

Now… all this talk about food is making me as hungry as a bear. Check out the Three Bean Salad with Honey Mustard Dressing and meet me back here to learn about more fantastic foods in the next chapter. But, first…

TASTY TIDBITS

- Identify the health-food junk-foods in your home (soy chips, soy energy bars, soy protein drinks, fake meats, soy yogurt, soy ice-cream, etc.) and toss into the garbage.
- You could substitute canned beans in any of the bean recipes (just try not to make a habit out of it!).
- Do not eat too many beans in one sitting unless, of course, you have strong digestion or live alone and have access to fresh air.
- Try a new bean or bean product (tofu, tempeh, miso) every week.

---

[13] http://www.mothering.com/sections/news_bulletins/august2005.html#soy

CHAPTER 5

IN THE PASTURE

Old MacDonald had a farm, and on his farm he had a variety of animals… to eat. Naturally-raised pastured animals provide food that is calorically rich and nutrient *dense*. This supplies a large dose of nutrition in a small amount, and enhances strength and vitality.

As a group animal foods (meat, poultry, eggs, fish, dairy) contain vitamin B2 (riboflavin), B3 (niacin), B5 (pantothenic), B6 (pyridoxine), B12 (cobalamin), selenium, calcium, zinc, iron, phosphorus, selenium, vitamin A, copper, riboflavin, amino acids, Vitamin D, choline, lutein, Vitamin K, iodine, essential fatty acids, protein, amino acids, magnesium and many other vitamins and minerals.

Animal meats and derivative products were traditionally health-promoting choices containing vital nutrients that can benefit the heart and reduce the risk of cancer.[14] Unfortunately, modern *mass* production of animals has led to many unhealthy factory-farming practices resulting in disease-promoting animal products instead.

Mass-produced animals are usually kept in unsanitary conditions that breed sickness; they are housed in cramped quarters that do not provide adequate exercise or a natural living environment. They are fed a

---

[14] http://www.whfoods.com/genpage.php?tname=foodspice&dbid=141#healthbenefits

steady diet of antibiotics to help stave off disease and keep them alive, and are given growth hormones so they produce more meat and milk.[15] [16] [17]

"Antibiotics keep animals healthy while they live in their own waste as they are fattened for slaughter. About 30 million cattle go to slaughter in the USA each year. With each getting about 300 milligrams of antibiotics daily in the final months before slaughter, they account for about half the antibiotic use in the nation." [18]

If my food has been overdosed with antibiotics then so have I. "You are what you eat," and "You are what your food eats, too." Factory farmed animals are fed a steady diet of drugs and kept alive (barely!) in horrible conditions with many sick and dying before they are slaughtered. What big-business factory farmers are doing to animals is inhumane and unhealthy for both the animal and the consumers of these products. Animals need to live a decent life: graze on food they're designed to eat, exercise in fields of grass, have access to sunshine, clean water, fresh air, and reproduce naturally.

I need to know that the animal I choose to consume has led a quality life before I will put any part of its energy inside my body. I know whatever the animal is subjected to I am subjected to second-hand. If the animal I eat is unhealthy, I risk becoming unhealthy. I would no more eat diseased corn than I would a diseased cow. Quality of life is imperative when choosing animal food, or any food for that matter.

---

[15] http://www.hsus.org/farm_animals/factory_farms/
[16] http://www.hfa.org/factory/
[17] http://www.organicconsumers.org/Toxic/animalfeed.cfm
[18] Antibiotic Resistance Has Feedlots Riding Herd On Food Chain, by Robert Davis, USA Today, Tuesday, June 15, 1999, p. 6D.

Energetically, most animal food (chicken, turkey, cow, venison, goat, sheep, buffalo, eggs, quail, pork, etc.) strengthens and *warms*, with fish and dairy being the exceptions. Fish strengthens and *cools* and most dairy products cool also.[19] Eating warm-blooded animals can create a feeling of inner warmth while cold-blooded animals like fish can create a cool sensation (like a York Peppermint Pattie!).

People often think that *meat* is carcinogenic, but that's simply not true. It's the quality of our meat and the way we cook it that determines whether or not it will contribute to ill health. If our meat is burned or cooked for long periods of time at very high temperatures it forms acrylamide (heterocyclic amines) that is cancer causing. With that in mind, it's best to eat meat rare or medium rare and not well done or burned to crisp. That doesn't mean you can never eat blackened, grilled or barbecued meat – it just means to eat that type of food much less often so your body is not under constant attack from carcinogens.

As mentioned, animal foods are dense with nutrients and energy; eating *too much* without utilizing the energy derived from them can congest the body, make the system sluggish, and contribute to disease. An important aspect to remember: when eating animal food (or any food, even plants too), "quantity changes quality." George Ohsawa, a food philosopher and pioneer in Macrobiotics (Natural Whole Foods Diet based on Traditional Chinese Medicine), coined that simple yet powerful phrase. Many foods from both the animal and vegetable kingdom are delicious, nutritious and health-promoting, but if eaten in *excess* could do more harm than good. How much to consume of each specific type of food, whether from plant or animal origin, depends on your physical body and the

---

[19] Energetics of Food, Steve Gagne, Spiral Sciences 1990, pp. 107-108

environment you live in. This information will be discussed in the chapter Climate Control. Right now, let's continue to take this one step at a time, one chapter at a time, one idea at a time. Information, like food, is easiest to digest in small amounts.

Until then, check out one of my favorite simple, quick and easy recipes, Terriyaki Salmon. Or browse the recipe section and pick one that appeals to you.

TASTY TIDBITS

- Products derived from animals are dense in nutrients.
- For the sake of your health (and the animal too) purchase naturally raised, organic, hormone and antibiotic free animal products.
- Use the Resource list in the back of this guide to find suppliers and stores that carry better quality animal products.
- Most animal meats create warmth in the body.
- Most fish creates coolness.
- Remember, "quantity changes quality" - don't eat *too much* of anything no matter how good it is for you!
- Give your eyes a rest between chapters and refuel your body with something delicious and nutritious from the recipe section in Part II.

CHAPTER 6
THE SEA INSIDE

The human body is made up mostly of water, as if we have a sea inside. To help us sustain a healthy internal liquid environment we *need* to eat foods that come from the water. An important substance from the ocean, integral to human health, is sea salt. "The one fact no one challenges is that the human body needs salt to function. Sodium is the main component of the body's extracellular fluids and it helps carry nutrients into the cells. Sodium also helps regulate other body functions, such as blood pressure and fluid volume, and sodium works on the lining of blood vessels to keep the pressure balance normal."[20] Humans have long revered the importance of salt. So much so in fact, that people were paid with it – hence the word "salary" is derived from the word salt.

Unrefined sea salt contains an abundance of minerals and trace minerals: potassium, phosphorous, iodine, magnesium, sulfur, zinc, magnesium, iron, manganese, copper, calcium, silicon, strontium, boron, fluourine, lithium, germanium, scandium, gallium, and at least fifty more! Good quality sea salt, with its minerals intact, is highly beneficial to health.

However, refined commercial table salt, which has been stripped of its many essential elements, upsets the body's natural balance and

---

[20] http://www.fda.gov/fdac/features/1997/797_salt.html

contributes to high blood pressure, heart disease, osteoporosis, weight gain, cancer and other maladies.[21] Iodized table salt (sodium chloride + iodine + other chemicals) is dangerous – it's missing the other minerals that make it balanced. If the salt we eat is stripped of nutrients and imbalanced, when we eat it, we'll become imbalanced, too.

I highly recommend you take all of the refined table salt, iodized salt, and kosher salt (it's not healthy for you, so it's not *really* kosher), and use it after the next heavy snowfall to melt ice on the sidewalk. At least there it can do some good. But, whatever you do…don't put that poison on your food! For better health, it's wise to season your food with a natural unrefined sea salt. There are many different brands to choose from: Lima, French Atlantic, Celtic, Muramoto, Si, Spirit of the Sea, and others. Unrefined sea salt can be purchased at any local health food store, gourmet market, mail order company, or online (the Resources page has all of this information for you).

Sea vegetables are another nutritious food from the ocean. Many cultures around the world have gleaned numerous health benefits from eating sea vegetables. One study at the University of California revealed that kelp may be the most important cancer-fighting component in the Asian diet.[22]

Vegetables from the sea, also known as "seaweed" contain high concentrations of calcium, iron, phosphorous, potassium, sodium, zinc, magnesium, copper, chromium, vitamin A, vitamin B1, vitamin B2, vitamin B3, vitamin B6, vitamin C, vitamin, E, manganese, iodine, and

[21] http://curezone.com/foods/salt/understanding_salt_and_sodium.htm
[22] ODE Magazine, September 2005, pg. 69

more. Sea vegetables contain alginic acid that binds with toxins in our body and allows their natural elimination.[23]

Energetically, sea vegetables are cooling and can help to counteract "hot" conditions in the body, such as inflammation, swelling, hot flashes, and high blood pressure. Like caviar, sea vegetables are an acquired taste. Thanks to the popularity of Japanese restaurants many people have broadened their palates to enjoy the delicious taste of sea vegetables. Those cute little rolls that you may have eaten at the local sushi bar are wrapped in a sea vegetable called Nori. Other sea vegetables include agar-agar, alaria, arame, dulse, hijiki, Irish moss, kelp, kombu, sea palm, and wakame. I believe eating mineral rich sea vegetables was one of the greatest contributors to healing my thyroid dysfunction, and enhancing my overall health.

A young female client in her mid-thirties had a terrible diet: pizza, iceberg lettuce salad and diet coke – no joke… that was it! I could see she was severely vitamin and mineral deficient and needed to improve her food choices. She told me that although she wanted to change her diet there was "no way" she was going to eat sea vegetables because they were "slimy and gross." I asked that she just try incorporating a tiny amount (two tablespoons) two times per week and become aware of what happens inside her body.

Three months into her improved way of eating, she said, "something happened and I'm craving seaweed like crazy. I can't seem to get enough of it! Is it okay if I eat it every day instead of just two times per week?" I told her to listen to her body and honor it, but to remember

---

[23] Cooking With Sea Vegetables, by Peter and Montse Bradford, Healing Arts Press 1985, 1988 pg. 13

that eating too many sea vegetables too often may not be healthy either. Sea vegetables are a nutrient rich food; we need only a small amount to aid the body's healing process and promote great health. She ate what she felt her body needed and eventually found the proper amount to sustain a functional internal system.

I know sea vegetables might be "foreign" for many of you, but check out some of the delicious sea-veggie recipes in this book and you too, may fall in love with their unique and special flavor.

TASTY TIDBITS

- Take your iodized table salt and either use it to melt snow or toss it into the garbage.
- Unrefined sea salt is better quality salt that benefits overall health.
- Sea vegetables are rich in minerals.
- Be adventurous, add a small amount of sea vegetables into your diet.
- Eating is a learned experience - if we can learn to like coffee, cigarettes and whiskey, we can learn to like a little seaweed too!

CHAPTER 7

NUTRITIOUS NUTS & SENSATIONAL SEEDS

I'm nuts about nuts! Nuts and seeds are a great source of protein, essential fatty acids, vitamin E, minerals, amino acids and carbohydrates. Externally, their hard shell protects them from the elements and keeps them fresh for extended periods of time. However, once shelled their healthful oils can become rancid due to oxidation (eek!). And, nuts that are roasted in poor quality oils at extremely high temperatures speeds up that oxidation process (double eek!). That means most store-bought nuts and seeds (in health food stores too) may already be rancid even before you open the can or jar! What's a nutty nut eater to do?

For better health, it's best to buy nuts and seeds still inside their shell, but that can be highly inconvenient; cracking them open can be time consuming. Even I do not have the desire to sit and crack open a bunch of nuts – it would probably drive me nuts! Instead, I buy raw nuts and seeds that have been shelled and packed in airtight containers or bags that help retain their freshness. If I'm shopping at a health food store that generally has a lot of "shopper traffic," I'll buy raw nuts from the bulk bins because they don't sit shelled for long periods of time. Raw nuts and seeds can be refrigerated to extend their shelf life.

You can either eat them raw or dry roast them on a low flame for ten to fifteen minutes on top of the stove in a pan, or inside the oven. I love both roasted and raw nuts, but there's something about roasted nuts that tastes more hearty and delicious to me. They're just plain yummy!

Nuts and seeds are a better snack choice than fat-free pretzels, crackers, chips, or highly sugared protein bars. The concentrated protein, fat and fiber in nuts and seeds keep the body satisfied for longer periods of time than most other snacks. According to the Harvard School of Nutrition, nuts and legumes could be eaten one to three times per day to create a healthy balanced diet.[24]

Energetically, nuts can grow entire trees. Stop and think about that for a moment. One little walnut can grow an entire tree – that's a tremendous amount of energy, so it's best to eat nuts in small quantities. It can be quite easy for me to sit down with an entire bag of nuts and pop handful after handful into my mouth, but if those nuts were inside their shell and I had to crack them open myself it would annoy the heck out of me, and I probably wouldn't eat many of them. With that in mind, I keep my quantity to as many as I would have the patience to crack open – probably one or two handfuls, but definitely *not* an entire bag. It also takes a large quantity of nuts and seeds to make peanut butter, almond butter, sesame tahini, pumpkin butter or any of the other nutty butters, so I won't have more than two or three tablespoons at one time (unless I have PMS, or am feeling emotional!). And, I always purchase natural nut and seed butters that don't contain the added sugar and hydrogenated oils that most commercial brands do. The beneficial oils in natural nut and seed butter can separate in the jar, and need to be mixed thoroughly – once combined, store inside the refrigerator and it won't separate again.

---

[24] http://www.hsph.harvard.edu/nutritionsource/pyramids.html

Dense with protein and fat, nuts and seeds can be highly satisfying and nutritious, but too many at one time can congest the digestive system and contribute to gas and bloating especially if they are not chewed well. I'm sure we've all seen what happens with peanuts if they are not chewed well. It's the same thing that happens with corn – the digestive system cannot break it down and it usually comes out looking the same way it went in. I apologize for the *gross* visual, but I had to make the point to remind you to chew your food; otherwise, it might just pass right through you.

The nuts and seeds category includes almonds, cashews, chestnuts, filberts, hazelnuts, peanuts, pecans, pine nuts, pistachios, walnuts, pumpkin seeds, sesame seeds, sunflower seeds, and many others.

When I have the time, I enjoy making my own trail mix. Trust me, there's a notable difference between home made trail mix and the pre-made mix from the store. Try it once and I'm sure you'll get hooked. Make a big enough batch to last about a month and keep it in a sealed container. Below is the recipe.

Happy Trails - Trail Mix

½ cup each raw walnuts and almonds

1 cup each raw sunflower and pumpkin seeds

Water

Tamari or shoyu (can buy in any health food store or Asian market)

½ cup raisins

½ cup dried cranberries

¼ cup non-dairy chocolate chips (a little bit of chocolate isn't going to hurt you!)

¼ cup dried shredded coconut

Place each variety of nut and seed in separate bowls. Keeping them separate helps retain individual flavors. Mix ¼ cup shoyu or tamari with 1 cup water. Coat nuts and seeds with liquid and marinate overnight or 6-8 hours. The following day discard the soaking water. Heat the oven to 200°or warm. Place nuts on a baking pan, and seeds on a separate baking pan (nuts take longer to roast than seeds). Bake until dry and crispy. The almonds and walnuts can bake for up to six or eight hours. The pumpkin and sunflower seeds three to five hours. Let the nuts and seeds cool and mix them with raisins, cranberries, chocolate chips and coconut. This trail mix makes a great movie snack or anytime snack. Happy crunching and munching!

TASTY TIDBITS

- Nuts and seeds are dense with protein, essential fatty acids, nutrients and energy.
- If roasted at extremely high temperatures in poor quality oils, nuts and seeds can become unhealthy.
- For better quality nuts and seeds buy them raw and dry roast them yourself.
- Buy natural nut and seed butters. When you get home, mix well before refrigerating to keep the healthful oils from separating.
- If you have children, purchase whole nuts and seeds still inside their shell, a nutcracker, and put your kids to work!
- One or two handfuls of nuts and seeds per day, chewed well, can benefit health.
- Nuts and seeds make great snacks.

CHAPTER 8

FABULOUS FRUITS

Fruit is succulent and sweet. No wonder Adam and Eve couldn't resist the temptation of that darn apple! Besides being delicious, fruit contains a rainbow of phytonutrients known as catechins, flavanoids, indoles, limonoids, lycopene, monterpenes, phenolic acid, quercitin, terpenes and others. Simply stated, without the unpronounceable scientific blah-blah, fruit nutrients are good for the prevention and healing of disease.

For all of the ladies out there, scientific research has discovered that blueberries and cranberries effectively help prevent urinary tract infections. These berries contain compounds called proanthocyanidins and condensed tanins that keep E. coli from attaching to the walls of the urinary tract.[25]

Energetically, fruit cools and cleanses, and can help chill out an *overheated* condition in the body. Too much internal heat can result from eating excessive amounts of meat and animal foods, spices, fried fatty foods, and by overloading the digestive system with too much food in general.

Fruit can be a great substitute for sugared treats if you are seeking to reduce the amount of refined sweets in your diet (cookies, pastries,

---

[25] Natural Health Magazine – p. 24 and New Life Magazine, July/August 1999.

candy, cake, artificial sweeteners, etc.). It's important to know that fruit is high in sugar (fructose), and eaten in excess does *not* promote health. Most people don't equate fruit with sugar and trouble can begin if fruit is overindulged.

I met a client who had a large, inoperable brain tumor. I asked her if she was eating excessive amounts of sugar or sugar substitutes, (artificial sweeteners have been linked with brain tumors[26]). She said, "I do *not* eat sugar." But, when I asked her about her fruit intake she told me she ate mangos and pineapple everyday for breakfast, bananas at lunch, and peaches and plums in the afternoon, and then more bananas throughout the day. This was far too much sugar for her body to handle, especially in the climate she was living. In a tropical environment all that sugary fruit might work because she'd be sweating out the sugar all day long, but in a temperate climate, especially during cold weather when we're all bundled up, sugar can wreak havoc on our system.

Eating what's appropriate for your specific climate is one of the greatest keys to creating vibrant health; it will be discussed in depth in the chapter Climate Control. But for now, keep in mind that fruit *always* tastes better, and is best for you, when it's in season. For example on a brisk Fall day after the apple harvest, a fresh, crisp apple will taste more delicious than if it is eaten in the middle of summer when it often has a mealy consistency. I'm sure we've all bitten into a mealy apple at one time or another – yuck! Trust me… things might have turned out much differently in the Garden of Eden had Adam and Eve tasted a bad apple. Eating fruit (and other food) in season will give you access to the freshest and most delicious tasting food.

---

[26] http://www.cnn.com/HEALTH/9611/18/aspartame/

Some tempting temperate climate fruits include apples, apricots, blackberries, blueberries, cantaloupe, cherries, cranberries, figs, grapes, honeydew, lemons, mulberries, nectarines, peaches, pears, plums, pomegranates, raisins, raspberries, strawberries, tangerines, watermelon, oranges, grapefruits and others.

A few of my favorite ways to eat fruit: dried cranberries on top of my oatmeal in the winter, cool Strawberry Sorbet during the hot summer or just munching on a crisp apple in the Fall. I also enjoy preserved fruit spreads on a slice of whole grain bread with a smear of almond or peanut butter. I purchase naturally sweetened jams. Most commercial jellies and jams on the market contain a lot of added sugars that I don't want inside my body. Fruit is sugar (fructose) and is usually sweet enough.

Check out some easy fruit recipes in the Delicious Desserts section to help satisfy your sweet tooth.

TASTY TIDBITS

- Sweet, succulent fruit is a great substitute for refined sweets like cookies, cakes, pastries, candy, etc.
- Fruit has a cooling effect on the body.
- Fruit contains sugar (fructose), so don't over do it.
- You could enjoy fruit as a simple snack or delicious dessert.
- For the most satisfying texture and flavor, eat fruit when it's in season.
- Grab a tempting apple, get yourself a partner, and have a great time… making the Autumn Apple Crisp, of course!

CHAPTER 9

PICKLE-ICIOUS FOODS

Have you ever wondered why pickles and fermented foods were traditionally presented on a plate of food? I never really thought about it either until I began making the connection between food and health. All cultures have used some type of pickle or other fermented food; in Japan there were takuan pickles, oshinko pickles and umeboshi plums; China had kimchee; in the Middle East they ate dill pickles, sour pickles and garlic pickles; in Germany it was sauerkraut; Russian people ate kefir and pickled cabbage; and people in the Mediterranean ate olives and yogurt.

Humans made pickles and fermented foods to preserve them, but important chemical reactions took place creating great health benefits in the process. Naturally fermented foods are considered probiotics and promote the growth of healthy bacteria in the intestines, increase overall nutrition of food, aid digestion, and support the immune system.[27] Probiotics are essential to good health, especially with the widespread abuse of antibiotics in modern society.

Antibiotics are prescribed for everything from colds to ear aches to toenail fungus, and if you think there's no need to worry about this problem because you haven't taken any, think again! As discussed in chapter 5, In the Pasture, the livestock we eat has been overdosed with

---

[27] http://www.mercola.com/2004/jan/3/fermented_foods.htm

antibiotics because they are living in unhealthy conditions and are chronically sick. If my food source has been overdosed with antibiotics, then I have been overdosed with antibiotics, too.

The problem with abusing antibiotics is that they enter the body like an atom bomb and wipe out all bacteria: the bad that cause infections, and the good needed to maintain healthy intestinal flora. Not only that, but after the antibiotic atom bomb detonates inside you there are mutant bacteria survivors. Yes, that's right! Mutant bacteria inside your body. Egads! If that mutant bacteria population outgrows the good bacteria (by abusing antibiotics and eating a crappy diet), serious problems like Chronic Fatigue Syndrome, Irritable Bowel Syndrome, Candida Yeast overgrowth, cancer and many other degenerative conditions can develop.

The natural probiotics found in fermented foods and traditionally pickled foods contain beneficial bacteria. "Sauerkraut eliminates disease-causing bad bacteria and reintroduces good bacteria such as Lactobacillus acidophilus. Such friendly bacteria, which are often destroyed by antibiotic residues in our food, are necessary for healthy digestion and proper elimination of waste products." [28]

Not all pickled foods are created equally. It's important to note that heating fermented food and pickles destroys beneficial bacteria and enzymes. Recolonizing the intestines with good intestinal flora begins with buying raw, unpasteurized, naturally fermented products that can be found in the refrigerated section of the nearest neighborhood health food store or other market. Unfortunately, modern foods pickled in vinegar,

---

[28] Source: "The Cultured Cabbage," by Klaus Kaufmann and Annelies Schoneck, Alive Books, 1997, p. 59.

sugar and iodized salt (not sea salt) just don't have the same healing effect on the body as good old fashioned salt brine pickles.

If you're feeling adventurous, you could make your own pickles. I haven't included any pickle recipes in this book because I'm not a pickle maker, but I'm certainly a pickle eater, so I shop at the health food store for my "good bacteria." If you want to make your own fermented foods check out these two books; Nourishing Traditions, By Sally Fallon and The Cultured Cabbage, by Klaus Kaufmann & Annelies Schoneck.

Try a small amount of some type of naturally fermented food with dinner (or a few times per week) to aid digestion of meals and reintroduce good bacteria into your body.

TASTY TIDBITS

- Most cultures around the world eat some type of pickled or naturally fermented food (miso, pickles, sauerkraut, yogurt, kefir, etc.).
- These foods are considered probiotics (good bacteria) and can enhance digestion.
- Purchase traditionally made raw unpasteurized pickles, cultured and fermented foods in the refrigerated section of your local health food store, specialty market or online – there is a Resources page in the back of this guide to help you locate products.
- If your digestion isn't good, don't get stuck in a pickle… just eat one.

CHAPTER 10

THE SKINNY ON FATS

Contrary to what I used to believe when I was trapped in a "dieting" mindset, the body needs good quality fat to thrive. Eating a non-fat or low fat diet, in the short-term can help cleanse the body and clear a congested system, but if continued for too long it can do more harm than good.

"A deficiency of fat can create a sensation of inner cold; body functions slow down for lack of warmth, and the tissues grow brittle."[29] Lack of fat actually slows metabolism and other bodily functions too. This is important to note, especially if you think eliminating fat will aid weight loss.

Fat lubricates the inside of the body and makes other functions operate smoothly... literally. I had a female client in her late thirties who was constantly constipated. She told me that she hadn't eaten any fat or oil in her diet for many years because she was afraid of gaining weight. I suggested she incorporate a little olive oil and organic butter in her cooking, and some cold-pressed flax oil on her salads. Putting a little fat into her food, combined with changing the quality of her overall diet, and chewing well, made her bowels finally get moving! As an added bonus,

---

[29] Food and Healing, by Annemarie Colbin, Random House 1986, pg 195.

she lost the nagging ten pounds that had weighed her down for many years while she was suffering through restrictive dieting.

Fats and oils are potent sources of energy and help assimilate fat-soluble vitamins like A, D, E, K, and minerals. Fat forms a protective layer around nerve tissues, enhances fluid metabolism, directs nutrients to the nervous system, and energizes and warms the body. And, fat makes food taste darn good and more satisfying. Better fats are essential for better health.

There are many different kinds of fat to choose from. Polyunsaturated fats are liquid at room temperature and sources include: sunflower, safflower, sesame, flax, walnut and pumpkin oils. These are rich in essential fatty acids, assist metabolic functions, and aid physical and mental flexibility.

Saturated fat is solid at room temperature. Sources of saturated fat are found primarily in animal foods: meat, dairy and eggs but also in a few plant foods like peanuts, coconuts, cottonseed and palm kernels. Over-consumption of poor quality saturated fat has been linked to heart disease, low tissue oxygenation, slow metabolism and other degenerative diseases. But, saturated animal fats can be especially healthy in cold environments, or during the winter months to help warm the body – this will be discussed in the Climate Control chapter. It may be a good idea to lighten up on saturated fats, but not to discard them entirely.

Monounsaturated fats are liquid at room temperature and solid in the refrigerator. Sources include: olive oil, almond and walnut oils. Monounsaturated fats can help lower cholesterol.

Essential Fatty Acids (omega 3's) are what most people eating a fast food, nutrient deficient, Standard American diet are lacking. These healthy fats include cold pressed unrefined and unsaturated vegetable oils like flax, borage, and primrose oils. These three oils should *never* be heated; they are fragile and can oxidize and become rancid very quickly. Other sources of EFA's include nuts, seeds, tuna, salmon, mackerel, sardines, halibut, sea bass and other fatty fish. EFA's increase the production of prostaglandins that regulate hormones, energy production, reproduction, fertility, immunity and communication among cells.

At last, we have come to the "ugly" fats paragraph. These are the fats you should avoid at all costs. Hydrogenated oils, partially hydrogenated oils, and trans-fats are a recipe for chronic illness! Hydrogenation is a process that turns vegetable oil that is normally liquid into solid fat that resembles butter. For the sake of your health, do NOT eat anything that *resembles* butter! If it's butter you're craving, eat good quality organic butter. Hydrogenated fat blocks essential fatty acid absorption, causes sexual dysfunction, create trans-fatty acids, high cholesterol, paralysis of the immune system, cancer, arteriosclerosis, diabetes, birth defects, obesity, sterility and much more.[30] [31]

Hydrogenated fats and trans-fats are lethal products! No joke. "I can't believe it's not butter" should be called "I can't believe it's not illegal!" Sources of hydrogenated oils include margarine, soy margarine, vegetable spreads, vegetable shortenings, and any of the products they are used in, including most refined and packaged foods (diet foods, cakes, pastries, cookies, cereals and others).

Oil and fat adds richness to food, but we need only small amounts. If your food is bland and boring, and you're not enjoying it, then it's not

---

[30] http://www.mercola.com/2000/jun/10/trans_fats.htm
[31] Fats that Heal Fats that Kill, Udo Erasmus, Alive Books 1986, pg 111

satisfying one of the most basic human desires – a pleasurable eating experience. The recipes in this book use good quality fats and oils to make food taste rich and delicious.

For better health, use small amounts of cold-pressed vegetable oils for healthy salad dressings (flax, borage, extra virgin olive oil, pumpkin, sesame and sunflower oils), and for frying or baking, use sesame oil, peanut oil, olive oil, grapeseed oil, and good old-fashioned butter.

TASTY TIDBITS

- Eating a non-fat diet can slow metabolism and inhibit absorption of vitamins and minerals.
- Good quality fats are a potent source of energy so you only need small amounts.
- Identify all the hydrogenated fats and partially hydrogenated fats and the products that contain them (margarine, packaged foods, cookies, snack foods, junk foods, etc.) and toss into the garbage - you may need a really big garbage can for this task.
- Don't be afraid to incorporate some better quality fats into your daily diet.
- The recipes in this book contain good fats – so start cooking your way to better health!

CHAPTER 11

SUGAR PLUM FAIRIES

The body *needs* sugar! I bet you'd never have thought I'd tell you something like that, but it's true. Glucose (sugar) is fuel for the body and mind, but overindulging in the sweet stuff can lead to serious ailments like diabetes, obesity, heart disease, tooth decay, pre-menstrual syndrome, memory loss (where the heck did I put those darn keys?), bone loss, weakened immune system and much more.[32] [33]

Our Standard American Diet (SAD), rich in fast foods and junk foods, is dangerously high in refined sugars that compromise health. Refined sugar can be defined as any "food" that has been stripped of its natural elements (vitamins, protein, fiber, minerals, fat). Sugar ingested in a highly refined state is absorbed directly into the blood stream, causing an immediate rush of energy. This "sugar high" sensation lifts us up, creating a temporary elevation, and then crashes us back down. Inevitably, we crave more sugar to lift us up again ensnaring us in a vicious cycle of extreme high and low energy fluctuations.

To metabolize sugar effectively the body will deplete its own supply of vitamins and minerals. Over time this weakens the immune

---

[32] http://www.hsph.harvard.edu/press/releases/press02152001.html
[33] Healing with Whole Foods, Paul Pitchford, North Atlantic Books 1993, pp 149-150.

system, contributes to depression, severe mood swings, an overly acidic condition, and many diseases.[34]

Cocaine, heroin and sugar are all made using a similar process; remove the vitamins, minerals and fiber from plants until the only thing left is a crystallized substance that is harmful to the body and mind. Excessive sugar abuse can most certainly be categorized as a drug addiction. If you don't think so, try it yourself or ask anyone who has ever tried to kick the sugar habit cold turkey. Many people suffer from withdrawal symptoms that include headache, insomnia, anxiety, edginess, anger, irritability and depression.

You may think you are not eating an abundance of sugar, but you probably are if you're eating highly refined and packaged convenience foods. Check out the ingredients on most processed foods and you may be surprised to discover sugar in almost everything. Sugar can be cleverly cloaked as dextrose, lactose, maltose, corn syrup, high fructose corn syrup, sorbitol, fructose, brown sugar (which is usually white sugar with molasses or artificial color added to make it brown), honey, sucrose, granulated cane juice, malt syrup and other dubious disguises.

The detrimental effects of sugar can be clearly seen in children. They have much *cleaner* bodies than adults, and haven't had a lifetime of sugar abuse to dull their senses. If we give children candy, chocolate or other sugary food, within a few moments they may become extremely hyper, unfocused, uncontrollable, throw temper tantrums, or perform an act of rage (lash out at siblings, friends, parents or others). Of course, I'm not *really* suggesting we perform this sugary experiment on our children. However, most of us do it every day.

---

[34] http://www.beyondhealth.com/sugar-poor-choice.htm

A closer look at the ingredients on some popular breakfast cereals for kids reveals the sugar content:

Kellogg's Apple Jacks: Corn, wheat and oat flour, **sugar,** salt, *confetti*, **corn syrup**, milled corn, dried apples, **apple juice concentrate,** cinnamon, sodium ascorbate and ascorbic acid, yellow #6, calcium phosphate, niacimide, zinc oxide, reduced iron, turmeric color, blue #1, pyridoxine hydrochloride, baking soda, riboflavin, vitamin A, red #40, BHT, folic acid, vitamin B12 and vitamin D.

The first three ingredients are refined flour products. Flour is a refined food that has a high glycemic index (changes to sugar rapidly in the body). The second ingredient is sugar. Among all the artificial colors and preservatives, there is something called "confetti." I wonder if this is a food substance or something they rake up from the floor after the parade and stick it in the cereal box! But, seriously, if you want to know why little Johnny has Attention Deficit Disorder it may be because he's starting the day with attention deficit foods.

Another popular breakfast cereal:

Captain Crunch: Corn flour, **sugar**, oat flour, **brown sugar**, *partially hydrogenated cottonseed oil*, salt, yellow #5, niacimide, reduced iron, zinc oxide, yellow #6, BHT, pyriodoxine hydrochloride, thiamine mononitrate, riboflavin, folic acid.

Remember the section on oils? Hydrogenated oils like *partially hydrogenated oil*, is one of the worst substances for the human body.

And, below is a quick and easy breakfast treat for the kiddies:

Pop Tarts: Filling: **Corn syrup, dextrose, high fructose corn syrup**, crackermeal, modified wheat starch, *partially hydrogenated soybean oil*, dried blueberries, dried grapes, citric acid, xanthan gum, natural and artificial blueberry flavors, soy lecithin, red #40, blue #2. Outside Coating: Enriched wheat flour, **sugar**, *partially hydrogenated soybean oil*, **corn syrup, dextrose, high fructose corn syrup**, salt, leavening, water, niacinamide, reduced iron, vitamin A palmitate, pyridoxine hydrochloride, riboflavin, thiamine hydrochloride, folic acid.

A word of advice, if you are seeking better health for you and your children, eating a box of Pop Tarts is not the way to find it. Do *not* give this product to your children, do *not* give it to your pets, and do *not* give it to your neighbors (unless your neighbors are really loud and obnoxious and you're trying to kill them!). Eating this sugary stuff once in a while is fine if you are in good health, but on a daily basis it could lead to long-term health troubles. I'm not going to sugarcoat it (pun intended here!) removing refined sugar from your diet can be difficult because it's in almost everything.

I am not suggesting you become overly rigid and eat a completely sugarless diet; small amounts of *good quality* sugar is fun to eat and delicious. Some better sugar sources and sweeteners include maple syrup, barley malt, brown rice syrup, honey, fruit and fruit juice, agave nectar, and granulated cane juice.

And, if you have the choice between poor quality sugar (white sugar, high fructose corn syrup, etc.), or artificial sweeteners, always go for the sugar. Trust me. Artificial sweeteners are exactly what the name implies… artificial. If you are seeking better health don't put anything fake inside your body – keep your food *real*. Many artificial sweeteners have been linked with cancer, gastrointestinal distress, shrunken thymus, enlarged liver and kidneys, multiple sclerosis, neurological disorders and overall poor health.[35]

In this Eating and Recipe Guide you have access to naturally sweetened treats that do not have a detrimental effect on your health and, quite possibly, may be good for you! If your sweet tooth is aching, jump to the Desserts section and make yourself the Brown Rice Crispy Treats – they're delicious.

TASTY TIDBITS

- The body needs sugar - glucose is fuel for your system.
- Overindulging in sugary foods can contribute to vitamin and mineral deficiencies, weak immune system, depression, many diseases and overall poor health.
- Switch to better sweeteners like maple syrup, honey, brown rice syrup, fruit juice and granulated cane juice.
- Most packaged foods (especially kid's cereals) contain poor quality sugars and crappy fats too – get into the habit of reading labels. Check the ingredients on the packaged foods in your kitchen pantry, and then toss the offending products into the garbage.
- Do *not* use artificial sweeteners. For the sake of your health discard any food or drinks that contain aspartame, sucralose, nutrasweet, saccharin, or other pseudo sugars.
- Instead of unhealthy breakfast treats, give the kiddies (and yourself) some good old-fashioned oatmeal with a splash of maple syrup, or organic eggs and whole grain bread with butter and naturally sweetened jam.

---

[35] http://www.sweetpoison.com/aspartame-sweeteners.html

CHAPTER 12

CLIMATE CONTROL

In the past twelve chapters you may have discovered some better quality foods to incorporate into your daily diet to improve your health. Now, more importantly, it's imperative to understand where, when and why to eat specific foods.

For centuries, humans mostly ate locally grown food. Like all other creatures on the planet, we ate what grew in our immediate surroundings. This way of eating ensured the greatest health potential and freshest food sources. All living things are closely related to their *environment* and are important in some way to the survival of the other. [36]

Unfortunately, modern technology has changed that natural way of eating. Today, every type of food is available at any time of the year regardless of where it's from. We even have access to food that doesn't grow anywhere near the climate we live in; this can be highly detrimental to our long-term health. Consistently eating foods out of climate, and out of season, leads to deterioration of health and inevitably, disease.

According to John Matsen, ND (Naturopathic Doctor), "All plants contain potassium. Generally, the more sun they're exposed to, the more potassium and sugar they contain. During the cold winter months, when you eat foods that are high in potassium and/or sugar (such as salad and

---

[36] http://www.blueplanetbiomes.org/world_biomes.htm

fruits), the high potassium and sugar levels alert your kidneys that you're out in the hot sun (because these foods grow in sunny climates), and that your skin must be making lots of vitamin D. Therefore, your kidneys don't activate vitamin D, and you don't absorb much calcium. This results in low calcium levels, forcing the body to take calcium from other sources such as bones, teeth and membranes, thus weakening those structures."[37]

For example, bananas are rich in potassium and sugar, and they grow in the tropics where it's hot and sunny year round. A banana is the perfect food for people living in a hot tropical climate where they will literally burn off that large dose of sugar all day long. But, if those bananas are shipped to Canada or New York City (where I live) they contain far too much sugar, potassium and other elements for my body to thrive during the fall and winter seasons. In addition, I'm usually bundled up under layers of clothing, a wool hat and cashmere scarf, and still *not* sweating as if I were in the tropics under the hot sun. The question is… if I eat that banana where is all of the excess sugar going if I'm *not* releasing it through my pores and sweat glands? That sugar is going to throw me off balance, weaken my immune system, and contribute to disease. Imagine that! All of those negative reactions from eating bananas. Don't' get me wrong, disease doesn't happen after eating one or two foods from another climate; it occurs from *consistently* eating foods that are not indigenous to your environment, weakening the body over time. There was a time when I used to eat at *least* one or two bananas a day, now I eat approximately one or two bananas a year. Big difference. I have a feeling after this book is published some banana farmers are probably going to want to put a banana bounty on my head! But, the truth, energetically,

---

[37] Better Nutrition Magazine, September 2004 pg. 30

scientifically, and intuitively, is that eating tropical foods in a temperate climate is a one-way ticket to poor health.

On the other hand, eating food that's appropriate at each time of year and according to climate can help keep the body strong and balanced. During the cold seasons, in a temperate climate, humans have traditionally added more animal food and salt to their diet. Animal food is energetically warming and has higher sodium than most plant foods. Sodium in the diet stimulates the kidneys to produce vitamin D, helping us absorb calcium when we have limited access to the sun.[38]

I cannot emphasize enough the importance, for the sake of your health, to eat food that grows in your area, or in a climate similar to the one you're living in. This is one of the most significant factors in figuring out what type of food, when to eat it, and how much of it you could consume to support your health.

The USDA food pyramid and many other diets neglect environmental factors or seasonality. With the absence of these essential components most diets and eating plans cannot promote lasting health, and eventually fail. According to many "healthy pyramids" we are advised to eat three to five servings of fruit per day regardless of our location, climate, or season. That clearly wouldn't work if you lived in a wintry environment. What do you think would happen to people living in Northern Canada, Siberia, Alaska, Greenland or Antarctica if they ate pineapple, watermelon and mangos three to five times per day? Do penguins living in Antarctica eat mangos? Of course not! The thought of penguins eating mangos may seem ridiculous, but it's no different than

---

[38]

http://www.eatingalive.com/monthlymatsen.php?matsencommentsmonth=matsencomme
nts0209.html&BeenSubmitted=TRUE&Submit=Enter

someone living in New York State, trudging home through the snow in February, carrying a bag full of mangos or other tropical fruits they bought at the grocery store. Uh-oh… now the mango farmers are going to be after me, too! The bottom line is eating foods outside of our climate is detrimental to health. It does *not* matter how much antioxidants or phytonutrients, fiber, or anything else there is in fruits and vegetables, if it's not indigenous to the environment you're living in, it may not benefit you, and can actually harm you. For your physical body to function optimally, it needs to be more closely aligned with the seasons and climate wherever you live. The climate of a region determines what plants will grow there, and what animals will inhabit it.[39]

The easiest way to get in touch with better food choices to promote your health is to discover what's available in your climate at specific times of the year. Take the time and go to a local farmer's market to observe what's being harvested in your area. Check out http://www.localharvest.org/ to locate organic farmer's markets, Community Supported Agriculture (CSA), Food Co-ops, regional/seasonal restaurants, and organic farms.

I belong to a CSA in New York City and love it! I have access to the freshest seasonal produce and animal products direct from the farmer weekly. The idea behind a CSA is that you, the consumer, literally buy a share of the harvest in the beginning of the year. The farmer invests your money to buy seeds, plant and tend the crops, and then brings fresh food (your return on investment) once or twice per week to a designated site for you to pick up. Whatever the farmer harvests during the growing season, you get a piece of the pie.

---

[39] http://www.blueplanetbiomes.org/climate.htm

This way of buying and eating food is highly cost effective, great for your body, and the environment, too. For example, I pay $395 (not including meat and eggs) for approximately twenty-four weeks of produce. That comes out to $17 per week for two bags of food that could include two onions, one bunch of carrots, broccoli, Swiss Chard, cabbage, five sweet red peppers, four frying peppers, three eggplants, two jalapeno peppers, butternut winter squash, one bunch of beets, fresh basil, eight to ten small potatoes, and two leeks (this is a sample week, the harvest varies each season). That's a large quantity of organic food for a small price. I could pay that same $17 (or more) for one meal and a cup of tea at a local restaurant.

Buying locally grown food will save you money. It also keeps the farmer employed and happy, and you're not paying for food to be shipped from all over the country, or all over the world. You save in many ways: promote your health, support your local community, and maintain the integrity of the environment at the same time. Plus, you could take the extra money you saved on groceries and shop for new clothes! It's a win, win, win situation.

Keep in mind that it's okay to eat food that's grown outside of your climate just try not to make it the *majority* of your diet. Clients often ask what they should eat while vacationing in other countries and climates. I advise them to be adventurous and taste the native, local cuisine; eat what the "old-timers" in the village eat (it's one of the reasons why they get to be old timers). If you are visiting a tropical environment leave the apples and pears behind and eat bananas and mangos for gosh sakes. *Always* eat the native food wherever you are, with one exception… if you are vacationing in Cannibal country don't eat the stew in the big black pot!

TASTY TIDBITS

- Figure out what type of climate you live in – temperate, tropical, sub-tropical, polar, etc. Go to http://www.blueplanetbiomes.org/ or your local library.

- For better health, eat foods that grow in your region of the world.

- Even though something is available in the supermarket year round doesn't necessarily mean it's good for you.

- Support your community, shop at local farmers markets, and you can enhance your health at the same time.

- Tropical fruits are most nourishing when eaten in a tropical climate.

CHAPTER 13

SEASONAL SUSTENANCE

To help you better understand what to eat and when to eat it, I've created some lists of foods that are generally available during each season in a temperate climate according to what the local farmers are harvesting in the Northeastern United States. These crops will vary according to area; North America is a temperate climate with environments that are dry (desert), cold (mountain regions, northern states) and warm (southern states).

You can use these lists as a beginner's guide to help create fully balanced delicious and nutritious meals. But, the key to obtaining long-term vibrant health is to eventually adjust your menus to incorporate foods growing in your specific region, whether you live in a tropical (South America and Central Africa, Central America, South and Southeast Asia, India, East Indies), dry (North Africa, Southeast Asia, Central Asia, India, Australia), temperate (North America, Western Europe, parts of the Mediterranean, East Asia, Eastern South America), cold (Canada, Central and Eastern Europe), or polar (Northern Canada, Artic, Greenland, Siberia, parts of Northeastern Europe) environment. Many areas around the globe fall into various climate categories.

The *easiest* way to discover which food grows in your area is go to the local farmer's market and take a look. There are farmers' markets all over the country and all over the world. I have the greatest respect for farmers. I know they are growing my food and without them, I'd be awfully hungry. So…hug a farmer when you see one.

This part of the book is interactive; I'd like you to grab a pen and scan the lists, highlighting foods you recognize. If a specific food is available in your environment begin using it in your meals. If something is unfamiliar, be adventurous and let yourself taste something new. You may be surprised to discover the variety of foods with which you can create better meals. The recipe section is chock full of ideas to help you make these seasonal foods taste absolutely delicious.

TEMPERATE CLIMATE PRODUCE

VEGETABLES

Spring	Early Summer	Late Summer	Fall
Asparagus	Arugula	Arugula	Beets
Baby Beets	Broccoli	Broccoli Rabe	Broccoli
Baby Carrots	Broccoli Rabe	Broccoli	Bok Choy
Bok Choy	Carrots	Brussel Sprouts	Brussel Sprouts
Chinese Cabbage	Celery	Burdock	Burdock
Dandelion	Chicory	Cabbage	Carrots
Greens	Collard Greens	Carrots	Cabbages
Dill	Corn	Celery	Cauliflower
Endive	Cucumbers	Chicory	Celery
Fennel	Escarole	Collard Greens	Celery Root
Fiddleheads	Eggplant	Corn	Daikon
Garlic Scape	Fiddleheads	Cucumbers	Eggplant
Green Beans	Green Beans	Escarole	Garlic
Herbs	Herbs	Eggplant	Ginger
Lettuces	Endive	Green Beans	Kale
Lemon Balm	Lettuces	Herbs	Leeks
Mizuna	Mustard Greens	Endive	Lotus Root
Mushrooms	Okra	Lettuces	Onions
Parsley	Peas	Mustard Greens	Parsley
Peas	Peppers	Onions	Parsnip
Radishes	Red Radishes	Peas	Potatoes
Scallions	Snow Peas	Peppers	Pumpkin
Shallots	Scallions	Red Radishes	Rutabaga
Spinach	Shallots	Snow Peas	Shallots
Sprouts	Spinach	Scallions	Spinach
Swiss Chard	Summer Squash	Spinach	Squash
Spring Onions	Swiss Chard	Summer Squash	Swiss Chard
Sugar Snap Peas	Tomato	Swiss Chard	Tomatillos
		Tomatillos	Turnips
		Tomato	Watercress
			Winter Squash

An abundance of food grows in a four-season temperate climate. Traditionally, the greatest harvest season is during the fall. It's a time to reap what has been sown throughout the year. Generally, vegetables do not grow through the winter under the snow, but roots, tubers, ground and round vegetables (onions, garlic, cabbages, carrots, parsnips, potatoes, winter squash, beets, etc.) and dark leafy greens (kale, collards, bok choy, etc.) that have been harvested in the late fall could be used throughout the cold months. You can get these vegetables in any local market or health food store.

It's important to remember that you could eat food from any season if you desire, just make the *majority* of your meals as seasonal as possible to achieve your greatest health potential. For example, in the wintertime I eat an occasional cucumber and tomato salad (summer foods) but it's not the main portion of my diet. In the cold weather I crave more animal protein and fat. As a matter of fact, as soon as the weather drops in New York (around November/December) I naturally crave Maple Glazed Duck and Hearty Roasted Winter Vegetables.

HERBS

Spring	Early Summer	Late Summer	Fall
Chives	Basil	Basil	Basil
Cilantro	Chives	Chives	Chives
Dill	Cilantro	Cilantro	Cilantro
Marjoram	Dill	Dill	Dill
Mint	Marjoram	Marjoram	Mint
Oregano	Mint	Mint	Oregano
Parsley	Oregano	Oregano	Parsley
Rosemary	Parsley	Parsley	Rosemary
Sage	Rosemary	Rosemary	Sage
Tarragon	Savory	Sage	Thyme
Thyme	Tarragon	Savory	
	Thyme	Tarragon	
		Thyme	

Herbs enhance the flavor of food, improve digestion, and are a healthful addition to any meal. I use fresh herbs throughout the spring, summer and fall. Generally, I use more dried herbs during the winter, but fresh parsley is a main staple in my kitchen all year round because it adds freshness and zing to my meals. Get to know herbs and use them in your cooking – try one new herb every week. If a recipe calls for an herb that you don't particularly like, change it. My recipes aren't meant to be stagnant. I want you to alter the recipes to your liking. Trust me, I won't mind if you switch around the ingredients and add things you enjoy. Between us working together we can create the most fantastic tasting meals!

FRUITS

Spring	Early Summer	Late Summer	Fall
Apples	Apricot	Apples	Apples
Rhubarb	Blueberries	Asian Pears	Asian Pears
	Cherries	Blackberries	Blackberries
	Currants	Blueberries	Chinese Pears
	Elderberries	Cranberries	Cranberries
	Gooseberries	Figs	Dried Fruits
	Melons	Grapes	Pears
	Mulberries	Melons	
	Nectarines	Nectarines	
	Peaches	Peaches	
	Plums	Pears	
	Raspberries	Plums	
	Strawberries	Pomegranate	
		Raspberries	
		Strawberries	

In a temperate climate the largest variety of fruit is harvested in the late summer. Fruit doesn't grow during the winter, but can still be enjoyed, especially if cooked with a little bit of salt to keep the potassium and sugar balanced. Winter is the best time of the year to eat fruit in the form of apple pies, cobblers, stewed pears, spiced cranberry relish, or pickled as people traditionally did during the cold season. Dried fruits are a good cold weather option. Fruit doesn't necessarily grow in the early spring either, but you could use leftover apples and pears from the fall harvest, and dried fruits as well. I use raisins all year round, but in the warm summer months fresh, cooling and juicy fruits like watermelon, plums and peaches are the ideal.

ANIMAL PRODUCTS

As far as animals go… it's the same concept. Eat the animals (and their products) that could thrive in your environment; cow, sheep, goat, rabbit, deer, chicken, turkey, duck, pheasant, lamb, buffalo, etc. Seasonally speaking, chicken or fish would be considered a good animal food in spring and summer while duck and pork would be considered a better winter choice (heartier meat, more fat). Saturated fat insulates and warms the body; that's why larger quantities of animal food are generally more desirable during cold weather and less so during the spring and hot summer when fruits and salads usually become the main fare.

Spring	Early Summer	Late Summer	Fall	Winter
Baby Lamb	Beef	Beef	Beef	Buffalo
Chicken	Chicken	Chicken	Buffalo	Beef
Eggs	Fish	Fish	Cheese	Cheese
Fish	Lamb	Lamb	Duck	Duck
Kefir	Pheasant	Pheasant	Fish	Fish
Yogurt	Rabbit	Pork	Lamb	Goat
	Shellfish	Rabbit	Pheasant	Lamb
		Shellfish	Pork	Moose
			Rabbit	Pheasant
			Turkey	Pork
			Venison	Rabbit
				Turkey
				Venison

If you live near the coastline or on an island, eat the fish and seafood found in the surrounding waters. If you live in the interior of the continent eat the fish from the lakes, streams, and ponds (if they are not polluted). Your daily diet is relevant to where you live. Once again, this doesn't mean that you should never eat outside of your environment... it just means be conscious of eating "most often" the foods indigenous to your area. Local eating is good for your health and for the entire world. For example, if you live in New York City, the cost of shipping coconuts from Costa Rica to New York by far exceeds the cost of buying a bushel of apples from a local farmers market. Less fossil fuel is used to transport local foods to you, thus having a better impact on our environment as a whole.

People often say to me, "I don't know what to eat because nothing grows in New York City. It is covered in concrete." Yes, New York and other major cities are covered in man-made materials but the surrounding environment supports a wide variety of plants and animals. Central Park in NYC is fertile ground for raspberries, blackberries, mulberries, apples, crabapples, lettuces, scallions, purslane, chickweed, sorrel, mushrooms, burdock root, walnuts and other edible plants.

The surrounding waters in New York and the five boroughs are home to flounder, fluke, mackerel, black fish, striped bass, eel, blue fish, porgy, wild Atlantic salmon, snapper, clams, mussels, crab, shrimp, tuna, shark, abandoned automobiles (!) and much more. New York State is inhabited by a wide variety of land animals, too: deer, rabbit, cow, sheep, lamb, goat, chicken, turkey, pheasant, pig, etc.

As mentioned in the previous chapter, discover what is available in your area by browsing a local farmers market or go to Localharvest.org and check out some of the farms in your area. Talk to the farmers – they would know what your immediate area could provide for you. Once you get the general idea of what is available in your region of the world you could create meals that can dramatically improve your health and help you to look better and feel better after every bite.

The tasty recipes in Part II will get you started eating better quality food. At the beginning of each recipe section are some general guidelines, tips and fun facts about the food you're going to cook. Get ready to eat your way, deliciously, to better health.

<u>TASTY TIDBITS</u>

- The seasonal food lists in this chapter are what is generally available in a temperate climate. And, the recipes in this guide were created with those specific foods in mind.
- Take note of the foods that are available in your area.
- If you don't know what grows in your environment, go to a local farmers market and do a little investigating.
- Check out www.localharvest.org to locate a farmers market, greenmarket, community supported agriculture (CSA), food co-op, or an organic, sustainable restaurant near you.
- For better health, change your food choices with each season.
- Be adventurous, try new foods and recipes.
- It's time to get into that kitchen and rattle those pots and pans!

PART II

BETTER FOOD RECIPES

SOUPS AND STARTERS

Creamy Broccoli Soup

Magical Miso Soup

Mushroom La Roux

Mighty Minestrone

Barley Mushroom Soup

Carrot Ginger Soup

Awesome Asparagus Soup

Pasta Fagiole

Heart Healthy Hummus

Baba Wawa Ganouj

Walnut Lentil Pate

Savory Stuffed Mushrooms

The key to using the recipes in Part II is flexibility. And, of course, practice! Every kitchen is different: from the pots and pans, type of stove, or the climate you live in (moisture in the air can affect recipes) – all of these intricacies contribute to the taste and quality of your finished product. Get into your kitchen, practice cooking, and you'll soon discover recipe results may vary according to the equipment you use and your personal environment. Be patient, follow the general guidelines, and be adaptable. Cook something once and decide if you need to alter the recipe in any way (more/less water, longer/shorter cooking time, lower/higher flame). Don't worry... I won't be offended if you change a recipe!

I cook on a gas stove using stainless steel pots and pans but have cooked in many homes that use electric stoves and other cookware (cast iron, glassware, non-stick, etc.). Whenever I ventured into other people's kitchens, the recipes required slight adjustments. Remember to be flexible; I want these recipes to work magnificently in your kitchen, not just my own.

Soups and Starters make great appetizers, but could be eaten as full meals or snacks, too. I sometimes have soup for breakfast or as a mid-afternoon treat. There is no specific time or place for any type of food. Whenever you feel like trying out a new recipe – go for it!

There is a glossary at the end of the recipe section to assist you with unfamiliar ingredients, and the Resources page will help you find them. Whenever possible, use the best quality foods: organic, locally grown, and seasonal. By consistently using better ingredients, your food will taste better and be better for you.

Now, let's cut out the chatter and start cooking!

Creamy Broccoli Soup (Sans The Cream!)

3 broccoli stalks, florets and
stems

2 red potatoes, cut into large
chunks

5 cups water or chicken stock

2 garlic cloves, peeled

2 tsp. Herbamare (herbed sea
salt) or 1 tsp. sea salt

Black pepper

Toasted pumpkin seeds

Bring all ingredients, except pumpkin seeds to a boil. Cover, lower flame
and simmer for 10-15 minutes. Remove vegetables with a slotted spoon
and puree in a blender or food processor. Add pureed vegetables back to
soup. Garnish with toasted pumpkin seeds. Serves four.

Magical Miso Soup

2 inches dried wakame sea
vegetable

5 cups water

6-7 shitake mushrooms caps,
sliced thin

6 ounces extra firm tofu, diced
into one inch cubes

2 heaping tbsp. unpasteurized
sweet white miso, diluted in a
small amount of water

2-3 scallions, minced (use both
white and green part of the
scallion)

Crumble wakame into water, add shitake mushrooms, tofu, and bring to a
boil. Cook for 4-5 minutes. Turn off the flame, and add diluted miso to
the soup (miso is a thick paste that needs to be thinned before adding it to
the soup; otherwise it remains a lump). Let the soup sit, covered, for 2-3
minutes. Garnish with scallions. Serves four.

Mushroom La Roux Soup

2 tbsp. olive oil or organic
   butter

2 tbsp. whole grain pastry flour

5 cups water

1 onion, peeled and cut into
   large chunks

2 cups cremini mushrooms

1 cup shitake mushrooms caps

1 tsp. sea salt (or to taste)

Black pepper

Parsley, minced (use both stem
   and top of parsley)

Sauté olive oil or butter in a pot on medium heat. Add two tbsp. flour and cook (stirring constantly) until butter and flour are combined. Slowly add water, stirring vigorously to break up any lumps. Add onion, mushrooms and salt, and bring to a boil. Cover and reduce flame to medium, cook for 10 minutes. Remove the mushrooms and onion with a slotted spoon and puree in a food processor or blender. Return pureed ingredients back to soup. Garnish with parsley. Serves four.

Mighty Minestrone Soup

1 tbsp. olive oil

2 garlic cloves, peeled and
   minced

1 small leek, cleaned and cut
   into ½ inch thick half moons

1 yellow summer squash, diced

1 zucchini, diced

2-3 leaves of swiss chard,
   chopped

2 cups cooked cannellini (white
   kidney) or great northern
   beans

5 cups water

2 bay leaves

1 tbsp. fresh basil or ½ tbsp.
   dried

¼ cup fresh parsley, minced

1 tbsp. tomato paste, diluted in
   a small amount of water

Sea Salt and Pepper to taste

½ cup quinoa pasta spirals or
   other pasta

Sauté garlic, leek, yellow summer squash and green zucchini for 2-3
minutes. Add swiss chard and cook for 1-2 minutes. Add beans, bay
leaves, water, tomato paste (dilute tomato paste in a small amount of water
before adding to soup), basil, parsley, salt, pepper and pasta. Bring to a
boil. Reduce flame, cover and simmer 8-10 minutes. Serves four.

Carrot Ginger Soup

10-12 carrots, diced

2 inches ginger, peeled

3 cups water

2 cups apple juice or cider

4-5 cloves, whole

½ tsp. sea salt

3-4 chives, minced

Bring all ingredients to a boil, except chives. Cover and cook on medium heat for 15 minutes or until carrots are soft. With a slotted spoon, remove carrots, ginger and cloves, and puree in a food processor or blender with one cup of soup broth. Add pureed ingredients back to soup. Garnish with fresh chives. Serves four.

Lentil Soup

1 tbsp. olive oil

1 onion, peeled and diced

2 garlic cloves, peeled and
   minced

2 carrots, diced

2 celery stalks, diced

1 tsp. cumin

½ tsp. coriander

½ tsp. sea salt

2 cups cooked lentils

4 cups water

¼ cup cilantro, minced

On a medium high heat, sauté onion and garlic for 2-3 minutes. Add carrots, celery, cumin, coriander and sea salt. Continue sautéing for 3-4 minutes. Add cooked lentils and water. Cover and cook for 10 minutes. Add cilantro and continue cooking for 1-2 minutes. Serves four.

Awesome Asparagus Soup

1 bunch asparagus

1 large leek, cut in half and
  cleaned

2 medium Yukon gold
  potatoes, chopped

4 cups water

1 tsp. sea salt

1 tbsp. dulse flakes

2 scallions, minced

Cut the woody bottoms off the asparagus shoots (about one inch) and discard. Place asparagus, leek, potatoes, water and sea salt into a pot. Bring to a boil, cover and cook on medium for 10 minutes. Remove vegetables and puree in a blender or food processor. Add back to the soup. Garnish with a sprinkle of dulse flakes and minced scallions. Serves four.

Pasta Fagiole

1 cup cannelini beans (white
kidney beans), soaked
overnight

2-3 bay leaves

3 cups water

5 cups chicken stock (or
vegetable stock, or water)

1 tbsp. olive oil

1 leek, cleaned and sliced into
thin moons

2-3 garlic cloves, peeled and
minced

1 large carrot, diced

1 celery root, peeled and diced

1 tsp. sea salt

1 tsp. dried rosemary

1 cup dry pasta spirals (quinoa,
spelt, kamut or other whole
grain pasta)

2 tbsp. parsley, minced

Discard bean soaking water. Add beans, bay leaves, and 3 cups water to a
pot and bring to a boil. Cover and reduce flame to simmer for 1¾ hours.
In a separate pot sauté leek and garlic for 2-3 minutes. Add carrots, celery
root, sea salt, dried rosemary, chicken stock, pasta and cooked beans.
Bring to boil, cover and cook on medium heat for 25-30 minutes. Add
parsley at the end of cooking. Serves six.

Heart Healthy Hummus

1 cup chickpeas, soaked
  overnight
3 cups water
1/3 cup tahini
2 garlic cloves, peeled and
  chopped

Juice of 1 lemon
1 tsp. ground cumin
½ tsp. ground coriander
Sea salt and pepper to taste

Discard soaking water from chickpeas. Add 3 cups fresh water and chickpeas to a pot. Bring to a boil, reduce flame, cover and simmer for 2½ hours or until chickpeas are soft (save some of the chickpea cooking water to thin the consistency of hummus). In a food processor add tahini, garlic, lemon, cumin, coriander, cooked chickpeas and salt and pepper. Puree until smooth and creamy, slowly adding chickpea cooking water to create desired consistency. Serves eight.

Baba Wawa Ganouj

1 large eggplant, cut in half
  lengthwise

Olive oil

2 tbsp. sesame tahini

Juice of 1 lemon

1 garlic clove, peeled and diced

1/8 tsp. sea salt

½ tsp. freshly ground black
  pepper

Dash of cayenne pepper

2 whole grain pitas, cut into
  eighths (or small triangles)

Preheat oven to 400°. Lightly coat eggplant with olive oil and place on a baking pan with the cut side down. Place in oven and cook 45 minutes or until eggplant is soft and shriveled. In a food processor add sesame tahini, lemon juice, garlic, sea salt, black pepper and a dash of cayenne. Scoop out the inside of the cooked eggplant (discard the skin) and add into the food processor. Pulse ingredients until mixed but not completely pureed. Use pita triangles for scooping the eggplant dip. Serves four.

Walnut Lentil Pate

1/3 cup roasted walnuts

1 tsp. dried basil

2 tbsp. olive oil

1 shallot, peeled and minced

¼ tsp. sea salt

2 cups cooked lentils

3 tbsp. balsamic vinegar

Whole grain crackers

Put walnuts, basil, olive oil, shallot, sea salt, cooked lentils (can use canned or leftover lentils) and balsamic vinegar into the food processor and blend until smooth and creamy. Spread on whole grain crackers. Serves six.

Savory Stuffed Mushrooms

1/3 cup + 1 tbsp. olive oil

1 onion, peeled and minced

¼ tsp. sea salt

1 cup fresh basil leaves

2 garlic cloves, peeled and
   chopped

¼ cup pine nuts

¼ cup grated parmigian cheese

1½ cups cooked short grain
   rice

16 mushrooms (baby bella or
   button)

Preheat oven to 350°. Remove mushroom stems from caps, and chop the stems finely. Leave the caps whole. Saute onion in 1 tbsp. olive oil. Add chopped mushroom stems and sea salt, cook until soft (about 5 minutes). In a food processor puree 1/3 cup olive oil, fresh basil, garlic, pine nuts and grated parmigian cheese – this is a simple pesto sauce. Combine cooked rice, sautéed onions and mushrooms, and pesto sauce. Place a spoonful of rice/pesto mixture into each mushroom. Lightly oil a baking pan. Place stuffed mushrooms in the pan and cook uncovered for 20-25 minutes. Serves four.

SIMPLE SALADS

Mesclun Greens & Ravishing Radishes with

Carrot Ginger Dressing

Crunchy Cabbage Salad with Sesame Maple Dressing

Simple Pressed Salad

Sweet & Spicy Slaw

Watercress Salad with Pomegranate Dressing

Baby Beet Salad

Et Tu Caesar Salad

Omega 3 Tuna Salad with Raspberry Vinaigrette

Spring Greens with Balsamic Vinaigrette

All of the salads and dressings in this section can be mixed and matched. If you discover a specific dressing you absolutely love, you could use it on any of the salads included here, or in any of the other salad recipes in the bean, grain or animal food sections. Feel free to be adventurous and switch recipes to satisfy *your* taste buds.

The majority of the recipes in this entire guide are balanced using the five flavors; sweet, sour, salty, bitter, and pungent, but the ingredients are certainly not set in stone. There's no stagnation in a creative kitchen. Recipes can change just like the weather, and just like us.

I use seasonal ingredients that I enjoy, but I want you to figure out the flavors and foods that are available in your environment, and best for you. The more you begin to appreciate the taste of your food, the more inclined you'll be to cook meals. And, when you cook for yourself you nourish your body intimately because your food literally touches you on the inside. Cooking for yourself can be the beginning of a great relationship as you learn to understand your physical body, and how to truly satisfy its needs.

Use these recipes as guidelines to create balanced dishes and then experiment with other ingredients and have some fun. Contrary to what your parents may have told you when you were growing up, I want you to "play with your food!"

Mesclun Greens And Ravishing Radishes With
Carrot/Ginger Dressing

1 bag Mesclun greens or other
   green lettuces
1 cucumber, peeled and sliced
   into thin rounds

4 red radishes, sliced thin
¼ cup grated daikon radish

Mix lettuce, cucumber and radishes. Serve topped with a dollop of
Carrot/Ginger Dressing. Yields two servings.

Carrot/Ginger Dressing

4-5 carrots, grated
2 tbsp. ginger, peeled and
   chopped
1 small onion, peeled and diced
1 tsp. stone-ground or Dijon
   mustard

2 tbsp. shoyu
¼ cup apple juice
¼ cup apple cider vinegar
1/3 cup olive oil
2 tbsp. toasted sesame oil
Water for consistency

Puree all ingredients in a blender or food processor until creamy. Add
water to achieve desired consistency.

Crunchy Cabbage Salad With
Sesame Maple Dressing

1 cup each finely chopped
  green and purple cabbage
1 cup grated carrots
1 green apple, cored and sliced
  thin

2-3 scallions, minced (use both
  whte and green part of
  scallion)
2 tbsp. toasted sesame seeds

Combine all ingredients in a large bowl and coat with **Sesame Maple dressing**. Marinate for two hours on the counter (covered), or overnight inside the refrigerator (marinating inside the refrigerator takes longer). Garnish with toasted sesame seeds. Serves four.

Sesame Maple Dressing

3 tbsp. shoyu or tamari
¼ cup toasted sesame oil
2 tbsp. pure maple syrup
  Juice of 1 lemon

1 tbsp. ginger juice (grate ginger
  and squeeze with your hand or
  in a cheese cloth to obtain
  juice)

This is one of my favorite dressings – I use it on everything. Combine all ingredients and enjoy!

Simple Pressed Salad

6-8 Chinese cabbage leaves,
    sliced thin (can substitute
    other cabbage)
2-3 red radishes, sliced thin
1 fresh fennel root, sliced thin
2 scallions, minced

1 carrot, cut into thin diagonals
1 tsp. sea salt
2 tbsp. cilantro, minced

Place all ingredients, except cilantro, in a mixing bowl and work the sea salt in with your hands. Work the sea salt into the vegetables by squeezing with your hands (this breaks down the tough cellulose fibers). Put the vegetables into a salad press and apply pressure for 45 minutes. If you do not have a salad press, put the ingredients in a large mixing bowl. Place a flat dinner plate on top of the vegetables, and then a heavy object (like a pot filled with water) on top of the plate. The pressure from the heavy object will press the vegetables. Let the vegetables press for one hour (less time is needed with an actual salad press). The vegetables will release water. Drain the water and discard. Garnish with minced cilantro. Serves four.

Sweet & Spicy Slaw

½ head of Chinese cabbage,
   sliced thin

2-3 scallions cut on thin
   diagonals

2 carrots, shredded or grated

2 tsp. sea salt

1/3 cup apple cider vinegar

1 tbsp. hot pepper sesame oil

3 tbsp. honey

¼ cup tahini

2 tbsp. shoyu

Combine vegetables in a large mixing bowl. Work the sea salt in with your hands (slightly crush the vegetables when working in the salt). Let sit for 40-45 minutes – you can apply pressure to maximize slaw consistency and the break down of cabbage (use the method in the Simple Pressed Salad recipe). Discard the water released from the vegetables. Mix apple cider vinegar, hot pepper sesame oil, honey, tahini and shoyu. Coat the vegetables and marinate for 45 minutes. Serves four.

Watercress Salad With
Pomegranate Dressing

1 bunch watercress

1 cup daikon radish, cut into
thick matchsticks

1 bunch sunflower sprouts

1 carrot, cut into thin
matchsticks

¼ cup pomegranate seeds

Rinse watercress and toss with daikon radish, sunflower sprouts, carrots and pomegranate seeds. To get pomegranate seeds, buy a whole pomegranate, and peel to reveal the beautiful crimson colored seeds. Marinate your salad with **Pomegranate Dressing** for 25 minutes, tossing occasionally. Serves four.

Pomegranate Dressing

1/3 cup olive oil

3 tbsp. pomegranate
concentrate (can buy in the
health food store or specialty
market)

1 tbsp. maple syrup

Juice of 2 limes

Sea salt and black pepper

If you can't find pomegranate concentrate you could substitute black cherry concentrate or cranberry concentrate. Whisk all ingredients together.

Baby Beet Salad

7-8 baby beets (baby beets are
small spring beets – you can
substitute regular sized
beets)

2 cups of water

½ onion, peeled and sliced into
thin crescents

2 tbsp. Fresh dill, minced or ½
tbsp. dried dill

Juice and zest of one lemon

¼ cup olive oil

Sea salt

Black Pepper

Bring beets and water to a boil. Reduce heat to medium and cook 35-40
minutes or until beets are soft. Remove beet skin and slice beets into ¼
inch half moons. The beet juice will turn your fingers and hands bright
red. To prevent this unsightly discoloration, you could wear dishwashing
gloves while cutting the beets…or you could have somebody else cut the
beets for you. Slice the onion into thin crescents. Combine beets with
onion. Whisk olive oil, lemon juice and zest, dill, sea salt and black
pepper. Marinate for 25-30 minutes. Serves four.

Et Tu, Caesar Salad

2 heads Romaine lettuce, ripped into bite sized pieces (discard hard lettuce bottom/stem)

1 red onion, peeled and sliced wafer thin

Caesar Salad Dressing

1 cup whole grain croutons (purchase croutons at the health food store or make your own by coating cubed bread pieces with olive oil and toasting in the oven at 300° for 10-15 minutes on a cookie sheet)

Mix salad ingredients and coat with **Caesar Salad dressing**. Top with whole grain croutons and toss gently.

Caesar Salad Dressing

½ cup olive oil

2-3 anchovy fillets

1 garlic clove, peeled and diced

Juice of 1 lemon

1 tbsp. prepared Dijon mustard

2 tbsp. red wine vinegar or balsamic vinegar

1 tbsp. granulated cane juice or molasses

1/3 cup freshly grated parmigian cheese

Combine ingredients in a food processor or blender until smooth and creamy.

Omega 3 Tuna Salad With
Raspberry Vinaigrette

1 small head red or green leaf
   lettuce, shredded (discard
   hard lettuce stem)
4-5 black olives, pitted and
   sliced thin

1 small red onion, peeled and
   diced
1 can tuna, packed in water

Mix ingredients in a bowl and combine with 1/3 cup **Raspberry Vinaigrette**.

Raspberry Vinaigrette

2 tbsp. raspberry jam
4 tbsp. apple cider vinegar
1/4 cup flax oil or olive oil

¼ tsp. sea salt
1 shake black pepper

Whisk all ingredients together.

Spring Greens With
Balsamic Vinaigrette

2-3 cups lemon sorrel (or other
   spring greens)

3 cups mesclun greens (or
   other baby lettuces)

¼ cup almonds, chopped

¼ cup raisins

2 tbsp. toasted pumpkin seeds

In a large bowl combine greens, almonds, raisins and toasted pumpkin seeds. Toss with **Balsamic Vinaigrette**.   Serves four.

Balsamic Vinaigrette

1/3 cup extra virgin olive oil

2 tbsp. apple cider vinegar

3 tbsp. balsamic vinegar

1½ tbsp. maple syrup

1 garlic clove, peeled and
   minced

1 tbsp. fresh basil, minced

1 tsp. fresh oregano, minced

¼ tsp. sea salt

Whisk all ingredients together.

VIVA VEGGIES

Steamed Greens & Tangy Tahini Dressing

Basic Blanched Veggies

Baked Summer Vegetables

Cruciferous Vegetables & Creamy Tahini Dressing

Garlicky Greens

Roasted Autumn Vegetables

Sauteed Swiss Chard & Zucchini

Curried Sweet Potatoes

Ratatouille

Leeks & Asparagus

Moo Shoo Vegetables & Spicy Plum Sauce

Some people may not appreciate vegetables, and I can understand why. Growing up, I was subjected to mushy, overcooked canned vegetables served in the NYC Public School system, and soggy peas and carrots in TV dinners, so it was easy to banish that food group from my plate. But, I've discovered that vegetables are versatile and flavorful, and can enhance the health benefits and taste of any meal when properly prepared.

A great way to enjoy cooked vegetables is to season them lightly and *not* overcook them. To ensure your veggies remain crisp and tasty, you could slightly undercook them because they will continue cooking after you remove them from the heat. Another way to keep vegetables perky is to blanch them in boiling water, and then quickly dip in cold water to stop the cooking process.

If a recipe uses a specific vegetable you don't particularly like, exchange it for something else. For example, if a recipe calls for parsnips and you're not fond of them, try another root vegetable like carrots or parsley root. There are many different vegetables to choose from and I'm sure you're bound to find a few you like, and may even grow to love. I suggest you be adventurous, try a new vegetable every week to help expand your palate and shrink your waistline at the same time.

Also, don't let a lack of ingredients stop you from trying a recipe. If you don't have the exact ingredients for a specific recipe, use what you do have and create something new and exciting. Remember to use seasonal and organic vegetables as often as possible to ensure the best tasting dishes.

Steamed Greens &
Tangy Tahini Dressing

1 bunch hearty greens (kale,   **Water**
  collards, etc.)

Clean the greens by rinsing under cool water. Rip or cut the leaves and stem into bite-sized pieces. Put water in the bottom of a pot with a metal steamer. Bring to a boil and add greens. Cover and steam for 3-5 minutes or until bright green. Top with **Tangy Tahini Dressing.** Serves four.

Tangy Tahini Dressing

3 heaping tbsp. sesame tahini   **2 tbsp. shoyu**

2 garlic cloves, peeled   **Juice and zest of 1 lemon**

1 tbsp. maple syrup   **1/3-1/2 cup water**

Put all ingredients except water into a food processor or blender. Puree until creamy. Add water slowly to obtain desired consistency. The more water you add, the thinner the dressing. This dressing will thicken in the refrigerator.

Basic Blanched Veggies

2 cups water

2 carrots, cut into ½ inch
   rounds

1 leek, cut in half lengthwise,
   cleaned and sliced on thin
   diagonals

3-4 Collard Greens, sliced thin

2-3 tbsp. toasted sunflower
   seeds (optional)

Bring water to a boil and add carrots for 1-2 minutes. Remove with a slotted spoon and let drain in a colander. Blanch leeks for 1-2 minutes. Remove leeks, drain, and repeat the process with collard greens for 2-3 minutes. Garnish with toasted sunflower seeds. Serves four.

Baked Summer Vegetables

2 patty pan squash or yellow
   summer squash, cut into ½
   inch rounds

1 zucchini, cut into ½ inch
   rounds

4-5 cherry tomatoes

1 tbsp. olive oil

2-3 pinches sea Salt

½ tbsp. fresh oregano minced

1 tbsp. fresh basil, minced

Preheat oven to 350°. Mix all ingredients in a large bowl, and then place into a baking pan. Bake uncovered for 30-35 minutes. Serves four.

Cruciferous Vegetables &
Creamy Tahini Dressing

½ head cauliflower, florets

2 cups broccoli florets

3-4 kale leaves (can substitute any other leafy green)

2 cups of water

Place a steamer basket into a pot with water. Place the leeks on the bottom, then cauliflower, broccoli, and kale on top. Bring water to a boil and steam veggies for 5-6 minutes. Top with your favorite dressing. I love the **Creamy Tahini**. Serves six.

Creamy Tahini Dressing

3 heaping tbsp. tahini

3 tbsp. shoyu

2 tbsp. umeboshi vinegar

½ bunch parsley (with stems)

4-5 scallions, white and green part

½-1 cup water

In a food processor or blender, puree tahini, shoyu, umeboshi vinegar, parsley and scallions. Slowly add water to achieve desired consistency.

Garlicky Greens

1-2 tsp. olive oil

2 garlic cloves, peeled and
   minced

2 tbsp. water

4-5 collard greens (or other
   dark leafy greens), cut into
   bite-sized pieces

Pinch of sea Salt

Add olive oil to a frying pan and sauté garlic on medium/high heat for 1-2 minutes. Add water, collard greens and a pinch of sea salt. Cover and steam for 3-4 minutes or until collards are bright green. Serves two.

Roasted Autumn Vegetables

2 medium sized delicata squash
   (can substitute 1 buttercup
   squash or other winter
   squash) deseeded and cut
   into two-inch thick chunks

1 large parsnip, chop into
   chunks

2 carrots, chop into chunks

Olive oil to coat

2-3 pinches sea salt

1 tbsp. fresh sage, minced

Preheat oven to 375°. To deseed the squash, cut in half lengthwise and use a spoon to pull out the seeds. There's no need to peel the squash – you can eat the skin of most winter squash (except spaghetti squash and carnival squash as the skin can remain quite hard). In a large mixing bowl drizzle squash, parsnips and carrots with olive oil, and season with sea salt and sage. Place vegetables into a baking pan and cover with aluminum foil. Cook for 45-50 minutes. Remove foil and continue cooking 15-20 minutes or until soft. Serves four.

Sautéed Swiss Chard And Zucchini

½ tbsp. Olive oil

1-2 garlic cloves, peeled and
minced

1 yellow summer squash, sliced
into thin rounds

1 green zucchini, sliced into
thin rounds

1 bunch swiss chard, cut into
bite-sized pieces

4-5 fresh basil leaves, minced

Sea Salt

1 tbsp. grated parmigian
cheese

On a medium high heat sauté garlic, zucchini, and squash in olive oil for
2-3 minutes. Add Swiss Chard leaves, fresh basil and a pinch of sea salt.
Cover and cook for 3-5 minutes, stirring occasionally. Sprinkle with
grated parmigian. Serves four.

Curried Sweet Potatoes

2 large sweet potatoes, diced
into 1 inch cubes (leave skin
on)

2 tbsp. olive oil

2-3 tsp. curry powder

Sea Salt

Preheat oven to 375°. In a large bowl combine sweet potato, olive oil,
curry, and sea salt, and coat evenly. Place potatoes in a baking pan, cover
and cook for 45-50 minutes. Uncover and continue cooking for 15-20
minutes. Serves four.

Ratatouille

2 tbsp. olive oil

1 onion, peeled and chopped into chunks

2 garlic cloves, peeled and minced

1 medium eggplant, cut into 1 inch pieces

2 zucchini, diced

2 tomatoes, deseeded and diced

1 red pepper, deseeded and diced

½ tbsp. dried basil

1 tsp. dried oregano

½ tsp. dried thyme

¼ tsp. sea salt

Dash of black pepper

On a medium/high heat sauté onion and garlic for 2-3 minutes. Add eggplant, zucchini, tomatoes, red pepper, dried herbs and salt and pepper. Reduce heat to medium/low, cover and cook for 35-40 minutes. Serves four.

Leeks And Asparagus

½ tbsp. olive oil

1 large leek

1 bunch asparagus

Sea salt

Black pepper

Lemon juice

Cut the leek in half, lengthwise, and clean the inside layers. Sometimes mud and sand can get stuck in there. Lay the leek flat and cut in thin diagonals, 1-2 inches wide. Chop off the woody bottom of the asparagus (about 1 inch from the bottom). Sauté leek on a medium/high heat, in olive oil for 2-3 minutes. Add asparagus and a pinch of sea salt and black pepper, cover and cook for 3-4 minutes. Squeeze fresh lemon on top of vegetables before serving. Serves four.

Moo Shoo Veggies & Spicy Plum Sauce

¼ cup water

1 onion, peeled and sliced thin

1 cup each, red and green cabbage, shredded

2 carrots, cut into thin matchsticks

2-3 button mushrooms, sliced thin

1 garlic clove, minced

2 eggs, scrambled and cut into thin strips (substitute cooked chicken cut into thin strips)

3 scallions, minced

Rice paper (buy in any Asian market)

Spicy Plum Sauce

Water saute onion for one minute. Add cabbage, carrots, mushrooms, and garlic. Cover and cook for 5-7 minutes. Add cooked egg strips and scallions. Soak rice paper in warm water until soft. Lay cooked vegetable mixture inside rice paper and top with **Spicy Plum Sauce**. Roll up and enjoy! Serves six.

Spicy Plum Sauce

2 tbsp. plum jam

3 tbsp. shoyu

1 tbsp. hot pepper sesame oil

2 tsp. grated ginger root

1 tbsp. molasses

½ cup water

2 tsp. kuzu or arrowroot + 2 tbsp. water

In a small pot on medium heat, combine all ingredients except kuzu. Dilute kuzu in water and add to pot. Cook for 2-3 minutes until sauce thickens slightly.

GREAT GRAINS

Basic Brown Rice

Summer Grains

Simple Short Grain Rice

Sizzlin' Stir Fried Rice and Veggies

Breakfast Porridge

Millet Mash

Ciao! Italian Rice Salad

Wild Rice and Zesty Orange Dressing

Quinoa, Aromatic Basil & Pine Nuts

Mellow Millet and Quinoa

Quintessential Quinoa Tabouli

Savory Kasha Pilaf

Primo Pasta Salad

Soba Noodles & Spicy Sesame Sauce

Sometimes, I reflect on past eating habits and can't believe my diet consisted primarily of highly refined grains (white bread, processed breakfast cereals, white rice, etc.). I practically lived on bagels – I don't know if it was a religious thing or a New York thing, but whatever it was… I'm glad it's history! Thank goodness for wholesome whole grains – they help me feel centered and balanced.

Whole grains are usually kept in large storage bins and should be rinsed to remove any dirt or dust particles. It's easy, just place the grains in a pot f water and swirl with your hand. Pour off the cloudy water and repeat one or two times until the water runs clear. For smaller grains like quinoa and millet, use a strainer with tight wire mesh and rinse under running water, otherwise you may lose half the grain down the drain!

As mentioned in Part I of this recipe guide, most grains should be soaked overnight or 8-24 hours. This starts the germination process making it easier to digest and absorb nutrients. If you forget to soak grains don't sweat it, they are still nourishing, delicious and highly nutritious – just don't forget to soak them on a regular basis. Traditional people soaked their grains and we should too.

Remember… digestion begins in the mouth; chewing thoroughly releases the carbohydrate-digesting enzyme ptyalin. Chew, chew, chew your food!

Basic Grain Recipes using one (1) cup of grain

GRAIN – 1 cup	WATER	TIME
Amaranth	2½-3 cups	20 minutes
Barley	3 cups	45-55 minutes
Brown Rice (short grain)	2 cups	45-50 minutes
Brown Rice (long grain)	1¾ cups	35-40 minutes
Buckwheat (Kasha)	2 cups	10-15 minutes
Kamut	3 cups	1½-2 hours
Millet	3 cups	25-30 minutes
Quinoa	2 cups	12-15 minutes
Spelt	3 cups	1- 1½ hours
Whole Oats	3 cups	2-3 hours

Rye and wheat are not on this whole grains cooking chart because they are more easily digested when sprouted or fermented (sourdough) and made into whole grain breads. I'm not an experienced bread maker so there aren't any bread recipes in this book. But, I do enjoy eating bread; I love sandwiches, poached eggs on top of toast, PBJ's (peanut butter and jelly sandwiches) and more. Some great quality breads can be purchased at your local health food market, Whole Foods, Trader Joes, Wild Oats, organic bakery, or other store. My favorite brands are Alvarado Street Bakery, Ezekial, Food For Life, and the organic breads at Le Pain Quotidien (a chain of organic bakery/eateries in the USA and abroad).

116

Basic Brown Basmati Rice

2 cups brown basmati rice,   3½ cups water
  soaked overnight   2 pinches sea salt

Discard grains soaking water. Bring rice and fresh water to a boil. Add two pinches sea salt (one pinch of sea salt for each cup of grain), cover and simmer 40-45 minutes. Yields six servings.

Summer Grains

1 cup quinoa, rinsed   2½ cups water
½ cup long grain rice, rinsed   Sea salt
½ cup of fresh corn kernels   ¼ cup chives, minced

Place quinoa, rice and corn in a pot with 2½ cups of water and bring to a boil. Add a pinch or two of sea salt. Cover and reduce flame to simmer for 40 minutes. Garnish with chives.

Simple Short Grain Rice

1 cup short grain brown rice, soaked overnight
2 cups water
Sea salt

Discard grains soaking water. Bring brown rice and 2 cups fresh water to a boil. Add a pinch of sea salt, lower flame to simmer, cover and cook for 45 minutes. Yields three servings.

Sizzlin' Stir Fried Rice And Vegetables

1 tbsp. toasted sesame oil

1 garlic clove, peeled and
minced

1 inch ginger root, peeled and
cut into matchsticks

½ cup water

1 onion, peeled and sliced into
thin half moons

2 carrots, cut on thin diagonals

¼ head cabbage, sliced thin

3-4 mushrooms, sliced thin

2 cups brown rice, cooked (can
use leftovers)

1 stalk broccoli, florets and
stem

8 ounces extra firm tofu, cubed
(can substitute cubed pieces
of cooked chicken, beef, or
pork)

2-3 tbsp. shoyu

1 tbsp. mirin (optional)

1 scallion, minced

On medium high heat, sauté garlic and ginger for one minute in toasted
sesame oil. Add water, onion, carrot, cabbage, mushrooms, and diced
broccoli stem, cover and cook for 3-5 minutes. Place cooked rice,
broccoli florets and cubed tofu on top of sautéed veggies and cover for 3-5
minutes. Add shoyu, mirin and scallions and cook for 2-3 minutes or until
broccoli is bright green. Yields four servings.

Breakfast Porridge

1 cup leftover brown rice

2 tbsp. rolled oats

1 cup water

2 tbsp. raisins

1-2 shakes of cinnamon

1 tbsp. toasted sunflower seeds

¼ cup rice milk, almond milk
  or other milk

1-2 tbsp. unhomogenized
  yogurt or kefir (optional)

Maple syrup

Bring leftover rice, rolled oats, water, raisins and cinnamon to a boil. Cover and simmer for 7-8 minutes, or until creamy. Top with toasted sunflower seeds or nuts. Add a little splash of almond milk or a dollop of natural yogurt or kefir, and maple syrup. Serves two.

Millet Mash

1 cup millet

3 cups water

½ head cauliflower florets +2
  tbsp. water

2 tbsp. butter or olive oil

1 onion, peeled and diced

Sea salt

Bring millet and water to a boil. Add a pinch of sea salt, cover and reduce flame to simmer for 25-30 minutes. While millet is cooking, sauté onion for 2-3 minutes on a medium flame. Add cauliflower florets to the pan, plus two tablespoons water. Cover and simmer for 7-10 minutes or until cauliflower is soft. Season with sea salt to taste. Combine cooked millet with cooked onion and cauliflower and mash until creamy. Serves six.

Ciao! Italian Rice Salad

1 cup water

1 red onion, peeled and diced

2 carrots, diced

1 yellow summer squash
(zucchini), diced

1 red pepper, diced

2-3 scallions, minced

3 cups long grain brown rice,
cooked

2 tbsp. parsley, minced

Italian dressing

Bring water to a boil. Drop onion into pot and blanch for 30 seconds. Remove with a slotted spoon and drain in a colander. Repeat the blanching process with carrots for 2-3 minutes, and zucchini for 30-60 seconds. Combine cooked vegetables, diced red pepper, scallions, cooked rice and parsley. Mix with **Italian Dressing**. Mangia! Serves four.

Italian Dressing

1/3 cup of olive oil

2 tbsp. balsamic vinegar

Juice and zest of 1 lemon

2 garlic cloves, peeled and
minced

2 tbsp. fresh basil, minced (or 2
tsp. if using dried)

1 tbsp. fresh oregano, minced
(1 tsp. if using dried)

¼ tsp. sea salt

1 shake of black pepper

Whisk ingredients together.

Wild Rice & Zesty Orange Dressing

1½ cups wild rice blend
   (purchase pre-mixed wild
   rice blend in the health food
   store or buy wehani, wild
   rice, basmati and others, and
   mix it yourself)

3 cups water

Sea salt

¼ cup roasted walnuts,
   chopped

1 granny smith apple, diced

½ cup diced roast turkey
   (substitute chicken or baked
   tofu)

¼ cup dried sweetened
   cranberries

1 stalk celery, diced

Bring rice and water to a boil. Add a pinch of sea salt, cover and simmer for 40 minutes. In a large bowl combine the cooked wild rice, walnuts, diced apple, diced roast turkey, cranberries and celery. Coat evenly with **Zesty Orange Dressing**. Yields four servings.

Zesty Orange Dressing

Juice and zest of one orange

1/3 cup olive oil

2 tbsp. balsamic vinegar

¼ cup maple syrup

¼ tsp. sea salt

Bring orange juice, zest, maple syrup, and balsamic vinegar to a boil. Cook on medium/high heat for 15 minutes, or until liquid is reduced by half. Combine with olive oil.

Quinoa, Aromatic Basil & Pine Nuts

1 cup quinoa, rinsed or soaked
  overnight

2 cups water

Pinch of sea salt

2-3 tbsp. pine nuts, lightly
  roasted

4-5 fresh basil leaves, minced

Bring quinoa and water to a boil. Reduce flame and add a pinch of sea salt. Cover and simmer 12-15 minutes. Toss in pine nuts and basil, and fluff with a fork. Serves four.

Mellow Millet And Quinoa

½ cup millet

1 cup quinoa

3 cups water

Sea salt

¼ cup cilantro, minced

Juice of 2 limes

¼ cup extra virgin olive oil

2 tbsp. shoyu

Bring millet, quinoa and water to a boil. Add a pinch of sea salt, cover and reduce flame to simmer. Cook 25-30 minutes. Mix cilantro, limejuice, olive oil and shoyu and combine with cooked grains. Serves six.

Quintessential Quinoa Tabouli

½ cup parsley chopped

4-5 scallions, chopped

¼ cup, fresh mint leaves

Juice of 1 lemon

1/3 cup extra virgin olive oil

2 garlic cloves, peeled and
  minced

¼ tsp. sea salt (or to taste)

3 cups quinoa, cooked

1 cucumber, peeled, deseeded
  and diced

1 tomato, deseeded and diced

In a food processor puree parsley, scallions, mint, lemon, olive oil, garlic and sea salt. In a large bowl, combine pureed mixture from the food processor with cooked quinoa, cucumber and tomato. Serves four.

Savory Kasha Pilaf

2 cups water

1 cup kasha (toasted
  buckwheat)

1 tbsp. olive oil or butter

1 medium onion, peeled and
  diced

4-5 cremini mushrooms, sliced
  thin

2 tsp. Herbamare or other
  herbed salt seasoning

Bring 2 cups of water to a boil. Add kasha, cover and reduce flame to simmer for 15 minutes. In a separate pan, sauté onion, mushroom and Herbamare on a medium high heat for 3-5 minutes. In a bowl mix cooked kasha with sautéed vegetables. Serves four.

Primo Pasta Salad

1 eight oz. package spelt or kamut spirals (or other whole grain pasta)

Water

1 red onion

1 bunch broccoli, florets

½ red pepper, deseeded and diced

3-4 sundried tomatoes, diced

5 black olives, pitted and sliced thin

2 links chicken sausage diced (optional)

¼ cup extra virgin olive oil

3 tbsp. white wine vinegar

1 garlic clove, peeled and minced

2 tbsp. fresh oregano, minced

1/8 tsp. sea salt

Cook pasta according to directions on package (should take between 8 and 10 minutes). In a separate pot bring one or two cups of water to a boil. Add onion and blanche for one minute. Remove with a slotted spoon and drain in a colander. Repeat blanching process with broccoli for 2-3 minutes or until bright green. In a large bowl combine blanched vegetables, cooked pasta, diced red pepper, sundried tomatoes, olives and chicken sausage. Whisk olive oil, white wine vinegar, garlic, oregano and sea salt. Coat the pasta and veggies with dressing. Serves six.

Soba Noodles & Spicy Sesame Sauce

1 eight oz. package soba
noodles (or other noodles)

1 cup sesame tahini

2 cloves garlic, peeled and
chopped

2 inches ginger, peeled and
chopped

¼ cup apple cider vinegar

¼ cup shoyu

3 tbsp. honey (or other liquid
sweetener)

2 tbsp. hot pepper sesame oil
(can use regular sesame oil)

1 pinch cayenne pepper

½ cup water

3 scallions, cut on thin
diagonals (use both white
and green part)

6-8 ounces baked tofu, cut into
½ inch cubes

1 tbsp. black sesame seeds,
toasted

Cook noodles according to directions on the package. In a food processor puree tahini, garlic, ginger, apple cider vinegar, shoyu, honey, hot pepper sesame oil and cayenne pepper. Add water to the food processor slowly to achieve desired consistency. In a large bowl combine cooked soba noodles, scallions, baked tofu and spicy sesame dressing. Garnish with black sesame seeds. Serves six.

BOUNTIFUL BEANS

Easy French Lentils and Vegetables

Basic Black Beans

Black Bean Burritos & Simple Salsa

Chickpeas and Capers

Rockin' Red Beans

Black-eyed Peas and Mustard Lemonette

Spiced Lentils and Sauteed Vegetables

Red Lentil Pate Nestled in Endive

Black Beans & Corn with Citrus Dressing

Hummus Wraps

BabyLima Bean Salad with Honey Mustard Dressing

Green Lentils and Winter Vegetables

White Bean and Arugula Salad

Three Bean Salad with Jalapeno Dressing

Pipin' Pinto Bean Chili

Tofu Chow Mein

Mushroom Medley & Tempeh with Miso Lime Sauce

Udon Noodles with Baked Tofu and Sesame Sauce

Cooked beans are savory, scrumptious, and versatile. You could interchange the beans in any recipe in this section just remember to adjust the cooking time. The cooking chart on the following page will guide you.

Dried beans do take time to prepare, but they are definitely worth the effort. To help save time in the kitchen, you could cook a large pot of beans once per week and store it in the refrigerator. That way you'll have enough leftovers to make spicy black bean burritos, colorful three bean salads, hearty bean soups, creamy bean pates, and more.

Lentils, adukis, and navy beans are small and do not require a long cooking time, but larger beans like garbanzo, pinto, anasazi, black beans, kidney and lima take more time. If you don't feel like cooking beans just yet, you could substitute canned beans in any of the recipes. Some better brands of canned beans that use good quality sea salt or kombu (sea vegetable) as their ingredients include Eden and Westbrae Natural. You can find these in your local health food store, other market, or online. The Resources page included in the back of this book will help you find everything you'll need.

Cooking chart is based on one (1) cup dried beans

BEAN (1 cup dried beans)	BOILING (water amount)	TIME
Aduki	2½ cups	50-55 minutes
Anasazi	2½ cups	1½ hours
Black Turtle Beans	2½ cups	1½-2 hours
Chickpeas	3- 3½ cups	2½-3 hours
Fava Beans	3 cups	1¼ hours
Kidney	3 cups	1¾ -2 hours
Lentils	2½ cups	45-55 minutes
Lima	2¼ cups	1½ hours
Navy	2¼ cups	1¼ hours
Pinto beans	2½ cups	1½-2 hours
Split Peas	3 cups	1 hour

Dried beans need to soaked be overnight or up to 24 hours. You could soak beans with a piece of kombu or kelp (sea vegetable); the natural glutamates in sea vegetables help tenderize beans. You could also soak in acidulated water (add vinegar), or just soak in plain water.

Discard beans soaking water and cook in fresh water. Bring to a boil and skim off and discard the foam that rises to the top of the pot in the beginning of cooking. Always wait until the beans are at least three quarters done before adding salt. Salting too early may contract the beans and keep them hard. Hard, undercooked beans could upset your digestive system. And, that in turn, may upset the people standing in your immediate vicinity.

Easy French Lentils & Vegetables

2 bay leaves

1 medium onion, peeled and
   diced

2 carrots, diced

2 celery stalks, diced

1 cup of French lentils (small
   greenish/black), soaked 8
   hours

2½ cups of water or beef stock

1 tbsp. fresh tarragon, minced
   or 1 tsp dried tarragon

2-3 tbsp. parsley, minced

½ tsp. sea salt

Discard lentils soaking water. Put bay leaves, onion, carrots, celery, lentils and fresh water or beef stock in a pot. Bring to a boil, cover, lower the flame and simmer for 40 minutes. Season with sea salt and tarragon and continue cooking for 15-20 minutes. Garnish with fresh parsley. Serves four.

Basic Black Beans

1 cup black beans, soaked
   overnight

2 bay leaves

2½ cups water

½ tsp. sea salt

Discard beans soaking water. Bring beans, bay leaves and fresh water to a rolling boil. Skim off foam that rises in the beginning of cooking and discard. Lower the flame, cover and simmer for 1 hour and 15 minutes. Add sea salt and continue cooking for 25-30 minutes or until beans are soft. Serves four. See the following recipe for a great idea on what to do with basic black beans.

Black Bean Burritos

1 tbsp. olive oil

1 onion, peeled and diced

2 garlic cloves, peeled and
  minced

1 yellow or red pepper,
  deseeded and diced

1 tsp. ground cumin

½ tsp. ground coriander

1-2 shakes cayenne pepper

1 cup cooked black beans
  (turtle beans)

¼ tsp. sea salt

2-3 tbsp. cilantro, minced

Sprouted whole wheat tortillas
  or whole grain burrito
  wrapper

Sauté onion and garlic for 1-2 minutes. Add yellow or red pepper, cumin, coriander and cayenne pepper. Cover and cook for 2-3 minutes. Add the cooked beans, sea salt and cilantro and continue cooking 5 minutes (if the pan gets a little dry you could add more oil or a little water). In a separate pan, warm the burrito wrapper on a low flame. Lay burrito wrapper flat, add some of the sautéed beans, and roll up. Put a healthy dollop of **Simple Summer Salsa** inside the burrito or on top. Serves four.

Simple Summer Salsa

½ cup cilantro

3 scallions, minced

2-3 tomatoes, deseeded

¼ tsp. Sea Salt

Juice of 1 lime

1 garlic clove, peeled and
  minced

1 jalapeno pepper, desseded
  and chopped

Pulse ingredients in food processor until you achieve desired consistency. I like this salsa a little chunky, so I pulse just a few times.

Chick Peas And Capers

1 cup chick peas, soaked 8-10
   hours with 3 inch piece of
   kombu
3 cups water
½ tsp. sea salt
1 cucumber, peeled, deseeded
   and diced
½ small red onion, peeled and
   sliced thin

3 tbsp. capers
1 tbsp. caper juice
1 tbsp. fresh dill or ½ tbsp.
   dried dill
Juice and zest of 1 lemon
1/3 cup extra virgin olive oil
1 tbsp. granulated cane juice or
   other sugar
Sea salt and black pepper

Discard chickpeas soaking water. Bring chickpeas, kombu and 3 cups of fresh water to a boil. Skim off foam that rises to the top. Lower flame to simmer, cover and cook for 2 hours. Add ½ tsp. sea salt and continue cooking for 30-45 minutes or until chickpeas are soft. Let chickpeas cool. In a bowl combine chickpeas, diced cucumber, onion and capers. Whisk lemon juice and zest, olive oil, sugar, caper juice, and dill. Season with sea salt and black pepper to taste. Marinate chickpea salad in dressing for 30 minutes, tossing occasionally. Serves six.

Rockin' Red Beans

1 cup kidney beans, soaked
   overnight

3 bay leaves

3 cups water

2 tbsp. olive oil

1 large onion, peeled and diced

2 garlic cloves, peeled and
   minced

2 stalks celery, diced

2 links organic andouille
   turkey sausage, diced

1 tomato, diced

½ tbsp. dried thyme

½ tbsp. dried oregano

1 tsp. allspice

1-2 shakes of cayenne pepper

½ tbsp. habanero sauce

½ tsp. black pepper

1 tsp. sea salt

Cooked brown rice

Discard beans soaking water. Bring beans, fresh water and bay leaves to a boil. Skim off and discard any foam that rises to the top. Reduce flame to simmer, cover and cook for 1½ hours. Remove ½ the beans and puree in a food processor or blender and then add back to the pot and continue cooking. In a separate pan sauté onion, garlic and celery for 5 minutes. Add turkey sausage, tomato, thyme oregano, allspice, habanero sauce, cayenne pepper, black pepper, and salt. Saute for 2-3 minutes. Add the sautéed vegetables to pot with the beans and cover and cook for 10 minutes. Lay beans on top of brown rice. Serves six.

Black Eyed Peas With Mustard Lemonette

1 cup black eyed peas, soaked
  overnight

2 bay leaves

3 cups water

1 tsp. sea salt

1 red onion, peeled and diced

2 carrots, diced

Discard beans soaking water. Bring black-eyed peas, bay leaves and 2 cups of fresh water to a boil. Cover and simmer for 50-55 minutes. Add sea salt and continue cooking for 20-25 minutes. In a separate pot, bring 1 cup of water to a boil. Drop in onion and blanch for 1 minute. Remove onion with a slotted spoon and drain in a colander. Repeat blanching with carrots. Mix black-eyed peas with vegetables and combine with **Mustard Lemonette**. Serves four.

Mustard Lemonette

1 tbsp. Dijon mustard

Juice of 1 lemon

¼ cup flax oil or extra virgin
  olive oil

3 tbsp. shoyu

1 tbsp. brown rice syrup or
  other sweetener

¼ cup of minced cilantro

Whisk ingredients together.

Spiced Lentils & Sautéed Vegetables

1 cup brown lentils

2 inches wakame sea vegetable

2½ cups of water

½ tsp. sea salt

1 tbsp. olive oil

2 garlic cloves, peeled and
   minced

1 large onion, diced

2-3 carrots, diced

2 celery stalks, diced

1 tsp. cumin

½ tsp. coriander

1 shake black pepper

Parsley, minced

Bring lentils, wakame and water to a boil. Reduce heat, cover and simmer for 45 minutes. Add sea salt and continue cooking for 10-15 minutes. In a separate pan, sauté garlic, onion, carrot, celery and spices until vegetables are soft, about 7-10 minutes. Combine lentils with sautéed vegetables. Garnish with parsley. Serves four.

Red Lentil Pate Nestled In Endive

1 cup red lentils

2 bay leaves

2 cups water

3 tbsp. shoyu

2 tbsp. balsamic vinegar

2 garlic cloves, peeled and
   minced

1 small onion, peeled and diced

3 tbsp. fresh basil, minced or 1
   tsp. dried basil

½ cup lightly roasted walnuts
   (roast in the oven for 12-15
   minutes at °325)

½ tsp. Black pepper

Endive

Bring lentils, water and bay leaves to a boil. Reduce flame, cover and simmer for 25-30 minutes or until the water is absorbed and lentils are creamy. Add the cooked lentils (remove bay leaves and discard), shoyu, balsamic vinegar, garlic, onion, basil, walnuts, and black pepper into a food processor or blender and puree. Separate endive leaves. Spoon pate into endive leaves. Serves six.

Black Beans & Corn With

Citrus Dressing

x 1 1/2

2 cups water

1 red onion, peeled and diced

1 cup fresh corn kernels

1 red pepper, deseeded and
  diced

2 cups cooked black turtle
  beans

2 tbsp. cilantro, minced

Sea Salt or Shoyu

In a pot, bring water to boil. Add onion and blanch for 30 seconds. Remove onion with a slotted spoon and drain in a colander. Repeat blanching with corn for 2-3 minutes. Mix cooked beans, corn, onions and diced red pepper in a bowl and combine with **Citrus Dressing**.

Citrus Dressing

1 garlic clove, peeled and
  minced

1/3 cup olive oil

2 tbsp. apple cider vinegar

Juice of 1 orange, plus 1 tsp.
  zest

Sea salt and black pepper to
  taste

Whisk all ingredients together.

Hummus Wraps

1 cup chick peas, soaked
overnight with kombu

3 cups water

2 heaping tbsp. sesame tahini

2 garlic cloves, peeled and
chopped

1 tsp. cumin

½ tsp. coriander

2-3 tbsp. shoyu

½ tsp. black pepper

Juice and zest of 1 lemon

1 package sprouted whole
grain burrito wraps or other
whole grain wraps

2 carrots, grated

1 cucumber, peeled and sliced
thin

Sunflower Sprouts, rinsed

Bring chickpeas, kombu and water to a boil. Skim off and discard any foam that rises to the top. Reduce flame and simmer for 2 hours 15 minutes. Season with sea salt and continue cooking for 30 minutes or until soft. In a food processor puree cooked beans, tahini, garlic, lemon and zest, cumin, shoyu, coriander and black pepper. Add leftover chickpea cooking water (or fresh water, or olive oil) to achieve desired hummus consistency. In a dry frying pan, heat whole grain wrap on a low flame. Lay wrap flat and add a couple of tablespoons of hummus, grated carrots and cucumber slices, and a bunch of sunflower sprouts. As you roll it up, tuck in the sides so the ingredients don't squish out. Serves six.

Baby Lima Bean Salad With
Honey Mustard Dressing

1 cup baby lima beans, soaked
  8-18 hours

2 cups water

2 bay leaves

1 tsp. sea salt

1 medium red onion, peeled
  and minced

2 carrots, diced

½ cup of fresh string beans,
  diced

¼ cup parsley, minced

Lima Beans have a soft skin and can easily turn to mush. To help them retain shape and texture, add salt at the beginning of cooking. Discard beans soaking water. Bring beans, 2 cups fresh water, ½ tsp. salt, and bay leaves to a boil. Skim off any foam that rises to the top and discard. Cover and reduce flame to simmer for 50 minutes. Add remaining ½ tsp. sea salt and cook an additional 20-25 minutes. In a separate pot bring 1 cup water to a boil and quickly blanch onions for 30 seconds. Remove with a slotted spoon and drain in a colander. Repeat with carrots for 3-4 minutes, and string beans for 1-2 minutes. In a large bowl, mix blanched vegetables with parsley and cooked lima beans. Combine with **Honey Mustard Dressing**. Serves four.

Honey Mustard Dressing

1 tbsp. prepared stone-ground
  mustard

3 tbsp. apple cider vinegar

1/3 cup extra virgin olive oil

1½ tbsp. honey

Sea Salt to taste

Whisk ingredients together.

Green Lentils & Winter Vegetables

1 large onion, peeled and diced

1 cup green lentils (can use
   black or brown too)

½ celeriac root (celery root),
   peeled and diced

2 carrots, diced

1 medium rutabaga, diced

1 parsnip, diced

½ cup winter squash, diced

2½ cups of water

1 tsp. dried thyme

½ tsp. sea salt

In a pot layer onion, lentils, celeriac, carrots, rutabaga, parsnip and winter squash. Add water and thyme, and bring to a boil. Cover and reduce flame to simmer for 45-50 minutes. Add sea salt and continue cooking for 15 minutes. Serves four.

White Bean & Arugula Salad

1 cup white beans (cannellini),
   soaked 8-18 hours

2 bay leaves

2½-3 cups water

2 garlic cloves, peeled and
   minced

1/4 cup extra virgin olive oil

2 tbsp. Balsamic vinegar

1 tbsp. Fresh oregano

Parsley, minced

2 tbsp. granulated cane juice

Sea Salt

Black Pepper

½ bunch arugula

Discard beans soaking water. Bring beans, bay leaves and fresh water to a boil. Cover, reduce flame and simmer 1½ hours. Add ½ tsp. sea salt and continue cooking for 25-30 minutes. Whisk garlic, olive oil, balsamic vinegar, granulated cane juice (sugar), oregano, sea salt and black pepper. Toss cooked beans with chopped arugula and dressing. Serves four.

Three Bean Salad With
Jammin' Jalapeno Dressing

2 cups water

1 red onion, peeled and diced

1 cup cauliflower florets

½ cup celery, diced

½ cup string beans, cut into
  one-inch pieces

1 cup black beans, cooked

½ cup chick peas, cooked

1 scallion, minced

Bring water to a boil. Add onion and blanch for 1 minute. Remove onion with a slotted spoon and let drain in a colander. Repeat blanching with cauliflower for 2-3 minutes, celery for 1 minute and string beans for 2 minutes. In a separate bowl, combine the blanched vegetables with cooked beans, minced scallion, and coat with **Jammin' Jalapeno Dressing**.

Jammin' Jalapeno Dressing

Juice of 4 limes

2 tsp. lime zest

1/3 cup sesame oil plus 1 tbsp.
  hot pepper sesame oil

2 tbsp. shoyu

1 jalapeno pepper, deseeded
  and minced

2 garlic cloves, peeled and
  minced

1/3 cup cilantro, minced

1 tbsp. honey or other
  sweetener

Be careful when chopping jalapenos that you do NOT touch your eyes, face, or any other body parts. Jalapenos are hot, and anything you touch will feel like it's on fire! Combine all the ingredients and enjoy.

142

Pipin' Pinto Bean Chili

1 cup pinto beans, soaked 8-10
  hours

3 cups water

2 tbsp. olive oil

1 large onion, peeled and diced

2 carrots, diced

2 stalks celery, diced

3 garlic cloves, peeled and
  minced

2 tsp. cumin

1 tsp. oregano

1 tsp. chili powder

1 tbsp. habanero or other hot
  sauce

1 tsp. sea salt

¼ cup of parsley, minced

½ cup raw milk cheddar
  cheese, grated

Discard beans soaking water. Bring beans and 3 cups fresh water to a
boil. Skim off any foam that rises to the top. Reduce flame, cover and
simmer for 1½ hours. Add 1 tsp. sea salt and continue cooking for ½
hour. In a separate pan sauté onion, carrot, celery, garlic, hot sauce and
spices for 5-7 minutes. Add sautéed vegetables to the cooked beans.
Cover and cook an additional 10 minutes. Mix in fresh parsley. Top with
grated cheddar cheese. Serves four.

Tofu Chow Mein

1 onion, peeled and cut into thin half moons

1 cup of celery, sliced on thin diagonals

½ head of Chinese cabbage, sliced thin

Sea salt

1 block of extra firm tofu, cut into 1inch cubes

1 tbsp. kuzu or arrowroot 2 tbsp. umeboshi vinegar

2 tbsp. shoyu

1 cup of chicken stock or water

2-3 scallions, minced

Cooked brown rice

Tofu is a quick and easy to prepare soybean product. On a high heat, water sauté (use ¼ cup water) onion, celery, Chinese cabbage and a pinch of sea salt for 3-5 minutes. Add tofu. Mix umeboshi vinegar, shoyu, chicken stock and kuzu together and add to the pan. Cover and cook 3-5 minutes or until the liquid turns clear and thickens. Ladle chow mein on top of cooked brown rice. Garnish with scallions. Serves four.

Mushroom Medley & Tempeh
With Miso Lime Sauce

1 package tempeh

2 tbsp. sesame oil

1 onion, peeled and sliced into thin crescents

6-7 fresh shitake mushrooms (discard the woody stems), sliced thin

½ cup of maitake mushrooms, sliced thin

1 head broccoli florets, and broccoli stems cut into ¼ inch diagonals

2 carrots cut into ¼ inch diagonals

¼ head of purple cabbage, sliced thin

3 tbsp. cilantro, minced

2 inches fresh ginger, peeled and minced

Juice of 2 limes

3 tbsp. White miso

½ cup of water

1 package of udon, soba or rice noodles (can substitute cooked rice)

Tempeh is a fermented soybean product – you can find it in any health food store or Asian Market. Dice tempeh into 1 inch cubes and sauté in 1 tbsp. sesame oil on medium heat for 15-20 minutes or until crispy. In a separate pan, use remaining 1 tbsp. sesame oil and sauté onion for 2-3 minutes. Add mushrooms, carrots, broccoli florets and stems, and cabbage. Cover and cook for 4-5 minutes. Add cooked tempeh to the sautéed vegetables. Mix cilantro, lime juice, miso and water and add that to the pan too. Cover and cook an additional 2-3 minutes. Follow the directions to cook noodles from the package of noodles (about 8-10 minutes in boiling water). Drain noodles. Ladle mushroom and tempeh with miso lime sauce on top of noodles. Serves four.

Udon Noodles With Baked Tofu
& Sesame Sauce

1 package udon noodles

½ cup sesame tahini

1 garlic clove, peeled and minced

2 inches of ginger, peeled and minced

¼ cup rice vinegar

¼ cup shoyu

¼ cup brown rice syrup or other sweetener

1 tbsp. hot pepper sesame oil

1 pinch cayenne pepper

½ cup of water (for consistency)

1 package baked tofu (teriyaki flavor), cut into ½ inch cubes

3 scallions, cut on thin diagonals

Tofu is a popular soybean product that comes pre-made in a wide variety of flavors and styles. Fresh tofu has a creamy consistency while baked tofu is chewy. Some flavorful baked tofu styles include teriyaki, thai, Italian, lemon pepper, and others. You can buy these in your local health food store or other store. Cook noodles according to directions package. Rinse cooked noodles with cool water, drain and set aside. In a food processor combine sesame tahini, garlic, ginger, rice vinegar, shoyu, rice syrup, and spicy sesame oil. Slowly add water to obtain desired consistency. Combine noodles and baked tofu with the Sesame sauce. Garnish with scallions.

SAVVY SEA VEGETABLES

Sea Veggies and Sweet Veggies

High Seas Hiziki Salad

Cooling Cucumber and Dulse Salad

Kombu with Winter Vegetables

Summer Sea Vegetable Salad with Mint Dressing

Crunchy Asian Slaw

Hiziki with Broccoli and Creamy Garlic Dressing

Sesame Burdock and Sea Vegetables

Arame with Presto Ginger Pesto

It's time to dive into some delicious sea vegetable recipes. That's right... I said delicious! Eating is a learned experience. Just like caviar, sea vegetables are an acquired taste.

Sea vegetables can be purchased at any health food store, Whole Foods, Wild Oats, Trader Joe's, or Asian market. If you don't have a market of that type in your area, you could order by mail or via the internet. Remember to use the Resources page in the back of this book to help you locate any foreign ingredients.

Sea vegetables are usually kept dried in plastic bags. If a recipe calls for ¼ cup hiziki – it means to use ¼ cup *dried* hiziki. Your sea vegetables will grow after you add water... just like a chia pet, only quicker. It takes about 5-15 minutes to reconstitute sea vegetables. In some recipes you will soak the sea vegetable before adding, and in others you'll just toss right in as they are. Follow the easy instructions to guide you toward creating successful sea veggie recipes.

Sea vegetables are mineral rich and a great side dish to any meal. Remember, we only need small amounts to satisfy nutritional needs.

Sea Veggies And Sweet Veggies

1 onion, peeled and cut into
   thin half moons

¼ cup arame, dried (soak for 5-
   10 minutes or until soft)

1 carrot, sliced into thin rounds

1 ear of fresh corn kernels

½ cup water

1 tbsp. toasted sesame oil

2 tbsp. shoyu

1 tbsp. brown rice syrup

2 scallions, minced

In a frying pan, lay onion, arame, carrots and corn on top of each other in that order. Cover with ½ cup water and cook on medium high heat for 15 minutes. Mix toasted sesame oil, shoyu and rice syrup and add to the pan. Cook for 5-10 minutes or until most of the liquid is absorbed. Garnish with scallions. Serves four.

High Seas Hiziki Salad

1 leek, cut lengthwise and then
   on thin diagonals

¼ cup dried hiziki, soaked in
   water for 10-15 minutes or
   until soft

3 celery stalks, diced

1 tsp. toasted sesame oil

3 tbsp. Shoyu

1 tbsp. mirin

½ tbsp. raw honey

½ cup water

2 tbsp. toasted sunflower seeds

Place leeks, hiziki, and celery into a pan. Mix the sesame oil, shoyu, mirin, honey and water and pour on top of hiziki and vegetables. Bring to boil, then lower to medium and cook 20-25 minutes. Garnish with sunflower seeds. Serves four.

Cooling Cucumber & Dulse Salad

3-4 cucumbers, peeled,
deseeded and sliced into half
moons

1 small red onion, peeled and
sliced into thin crescents

1 lettuce head, shredded

¼ cup fresh orange juice and 1
tsp. orange zest (grated
orange peel)

1 tbsp. granulated cane juice

1 tbsp. dulse flakes

Mix cucumber, onion and lettuce. Combine orange juice, and granulated cane juice. Coat salad and marinate at least 15-20 minutes. Garnish with dulse flakes. Serves four.

Kombu & Winter Vegetables

3 inches of dried kombu,
soaked and sliced matchstick
thin

1 onion, peeled and cut into
thin crescents

2 cups winter squash, cubed
(buttercup, kabocha,
butternut, etc.)

2 parsnips, cut into ½ inch
rounds

½ cup water

Shoyu

2 tbsp. parsley, minced

Place kombu, onion, squash and parsnip in a pan with water. Bring to a boil and cover. Lower flame to medium and cook for 20-25 minutes. Add a couple of drops of shoyu (not more than ½ tbsp.) and continue cooking until all the liquid has been absorbed. Garnish with fresh parsley. Serves four.

Summer Sea Vegetable Salad With Mint Dressing

½ cup dried arame, soaked

1 cup water

1 large red onion, diced

2 ears fresh corn (kernels removed from the cob)

1 cucumber, peeled, deseeded and diced

½ red pepper, deseeded and diced

5-6 fresh mint leaves, minced

3-4 tbsp. flax oil

Juice and zest of one lemon

1 tbsp. honey or other sweetener

Sea salt and black pepper to taste

Bring water and arame to a boil. Cover and reduce heat to medium for 15 minutes. Remove arame and drain in a colander. In a large bowl combine red onion, corn, cucumber, red pepper and cooked arame. Whisk flax oil, lemon juice and zest, minced mint leaves, honey, sea salt and black pepper. Marinate for 30-35 minutes or overnight in the refrigerator. Serves four.

Crunchy Asian Slaw

¼ cup arame, soaked

½ head purple cabbage, shredded

2 carrots, cut into matchsticks

1 cup water

¼ cup frozen edamame beans

3 tbsp. apple cider vinegar

4 tbsp. toasted sesame oil

1½ tbsp. honey or other sweetener

3 tbsp. shoyu

1 tbsp. ginger juice (finely grate ginger and squeeze with your hand or in a cheese cloth)

Cook arame in water, on a high heat for 10-15 minutes. While arame is cooking, finely shred the cabbage either in a food processor or use the wide holes on a cheese grater. Cut carrots into thin matchsticks or shred in the food processor. Drain the cooked arame and combine with the cabbage and carrots in a large bowl. Steam edamame beans according to directions on the package. Whisk apple cider vinegar, toasted sesame oil, honey, sea salt and ginger juice. Coat slaw evenly and marinate in refrigerator for 3-4 hours or overnight. Toss occasionally. Serves six.

Hijiki With Broccoli &
Creamy Garlic Dressing

2 cups water

2 cups broccoli, florets and
  stems (peel and dice the
  stems)

¼ cup hijiki, soaked

½ cup shredded beets (can use
  a cheese grater or food
  processor)

Bring water to a boil, add broccoli stems and cook until bright green or 2-3 minutes. Remove stems with a slotted spoon and drain in a colander. Repeat with broccoli florets for 1-2 minutes. Add hijiki to the water and cook for 15 minutes. Combine with **Creamy Garlic Dressing** and garnish with grated beets.

Creamy Garlic Dressing

3 tbsp. Tahini

¼ bunch of parsley

3-4 scallions

2 garlic cloves, peeled and
  minced

2 tbsp. umeboshi vinegar

1 tbsp. shoyu

½-1 cup water

Combine ingredients in a food processor and slowly add water to achieve desired consistency.

Sesame Burdock & Sea Vegetables

2-3 medium sized burdock
  roots, washed and cut on thin
  diagonals (do not peel the
  burdock – just scrub it clean)
2 carrots, cut on thin diagonals
¼ cup hiziki, soaked
1 tbsp. maple syrup

2 tbsp. shoyu
½ tbsp. mirin
½ cup water
2 tbsp. toasted sesame seeds

Put burdock, carrots and hiziki in a frying pan, in that order (burdock on the bottom, hiziki on top). Mix maple syrup, shoyu, mirin, and water, and pour into the pan. Bring to a boil, cover and cook on medium/low heat for 25-30 minutes or until liquid is absorbed and burdock is soft. Toss burdock, carrots and hiziki with toasted sesame seeds. Serves four.

Arame With Presto Ginger Pesto

1 cup water

2-3 carrots, cut into thin
   matchsticks

½ head cauliflower florets

¼ cup hiziki, soaked

1 red bell pepper, deseeded and
   diced

Bring water to a boil and blanch carrots for 2-3 minutes. Remove with a slotted spoon and drain in a colander. Repeat blanching with cauliflower for 3-4 minutes and drain in a colander. Add arame to the blanching water, cover and simmer for 10 minutes. Drain arame and combine in a mixing bowl with carrots, cauliflower and diced red pepper. Coat with **Presto Ginger Pesto**. Serves four.

Presto Ginger Pesto

2 inches ginger, peeled and
   sliced thin

¼ bunch cilantro, rinsed

½ cup pine nuts

2 tbsp. shoyu

1 garlic clove, peeled and
   minced

2 tbsp. sweet white miso

1/3 cup olive oil

½ - 1 cup water

Combine all ingredients, except water, in a food processor. Slowly add water to achieve desired consistency.

156

FISH TALES

One Pot Winter Stew

Pasta Putanesca

Super Salmon and Creamy Corn Bisque

Egg Drop Shrimp Soup

Shrimp with Pungent Plum Sauce

White Fish and Winter Veggie Stew

Creamy Cod Chowder

Terriyaki Salmon

Roasted Halibut with Miso Ginger Sauce

Salmon Croquettes with Dill Sauce

Tasty Tuna Burgers with Homemade Wasabi Mayonnaise

Simple Shrimp & Soba

When buying fish always purchase the best quality, preferably wild, and caught in waters that surround your area; streams, lakes, ponds, and oceans. It's okay to eat fish from other parts of the world, but for better health, most often stick to the fish caught in your immediate vicinity. Unless, of course, you live downstream from a nuclear power plant – fish that glow in the dark and have three or more eyes are not considered healthy choices.

As with all the recipes in this guide, you can alter the ingredients to your liking. If there is a particular fish you don't enjoy, change the recipe to include one that you do. Keep in mind the size and density of the fish and it will help you alter the cooking time. For example, if salmon is the ingredient I've provided, but you would prefer sole, keep in mind that salmon is a dense, fatty fish and needs longer cooking time than a light flaky sole. Measure the fish at its thickest part and cook approximately ten minutes per inch of thickness. If you don't have a ruler you could use your index finger - from the tip of your finger to the first knuckle is approximately one inch.

Some tips for buying fish; use your senses. Look at it. Fish should be clean and firm. If the fish is old, its skin and eyes may look milky, dull or slimy, and the fleshy area may have many cracks and crevices running through it. When the fishmonger isn't looking (!), touch the fish if you can – press into the flesh with one of your fingers (first make sure your finger is clean). The flesh should be firm, not mushy, and you should *not* be able to leave a fingerprint or indentation. And, lastly, smell that darn fish – take a good whiff. Believe it or not, if a fish smells "fishy" like a polluted bay at low tide, it's not a good sign. Fish should smell like the ocean: clean and fresh.

One Pot Winter Stew

6 cups water

1 inch ginger, peeled and cut into matchsticks

½ leek, cleaned and cut on thin diagonals

2 carrots, cut on thick diagonals

¼ cup winter squash, sliced thin

4-5 shitake mushrooms, sliced thin

8-12 ounces striped bass, skin removed and diced into chunks

1 cup broccoli florets and stem (peel stem and slice into thin rounds)

2-3 kale leaves cut or ripped into bite sized pieces

4 tbsp. sweet white miso

2 cups leftover grain (brown rice, noodles, etc.)

Watercress

Bring water, ginger, leek, carrots, squash, and shitake mushrooms to a boil. Reduce flame and simmer 5-7 minutes. Add striped bass and cook 4-5 minutes. Add broccoli stems and florets, and kale. Cover and cook 2-3 minutes. Dilute miso in a small amount of water and add to the soup. Add leftover grain or noodles and continue cooking for 2-3 minutes. Ladle into bowls and garnish with a sprig or two of fresh watercress. Serves four.

Pasta Putanesca

1 package whole grain pasta
(quinoa, spelt, whole wheat,
etc.)

3-4 anchovies (jarred or
canned)

3 garlic cloves, peeled and
minced

2 tbsp. Olive oil

1 tbsp. tomato paste

½ cup water

1 red onion, peeled, cut in half
and sliced into thin crescents

½ head cauliflower, florets

6-7 pitted black olives, sliced
thin

2 tbsp. Capers

3 tbsp. fresh basil, minced (or
1tsp. dried basil)

Sea salt

1/3 cup grated parmigian
cheese

Cook pasta according to directions on package. While pasta is cooking, in a separate pan, sauté anchovies, garlic and onion in olive oil for 2-3 minutes. Combine tomato paste and water, and add to the frying pan. Add cauliflower florets, capers, basil, olives and a pinch of sea salt. Cover and cook on medium heat until cauliflower is soft but not overcooked (5-7 minutes). Drain cooked pasta. Pour vegetables and sauce over pasta. Garnish with grated cheese. Serves four.

Super Salmon & Creamy Corn Bisque

1 red potato, cut into thick
    chunks

2 cups fresh or frozen corn
    kernels

1 onion, peeled and diced

1 tsp. sea salt

5 cups water

8 ounces wild salmon, diced
    (skinless)

3 tbsp. chives, minced

Bring potato, corn, onion, salt and water to a boil. Cover and cook on medium heat for 10 minutes. Remove ½ the vegetables and puree in a blender or food processor. Add pureed vegetables back to soup, and fish too. Cover and cook on a low heat for 5-7 minutes. Garnish with chives.

Egg Drop Shrimp Soup

4 cups chicken stock

½ pound small shrimp, peeled

4 scallions, minced

Sea salt to taste

½ tsp. black pepper

1 tbsp. Kuzu

1 egg, beaten

Bring stock to a boil. Add shrimp, sea salt, black pepper and scallions. Simmer 2-3 minutes. Slowly add beaten egg to the soup while stirring in one direction. Shut off heat and let sit for one minute. Serves three.

Shrimp With Pungent Plum Sauce

¼ cup water

1 red onion, sliced thin

2 heads broccoli, florets and
    stems (cut stems on thin
    diagonals)

1 carrot, cut on thin diagonals

½ pound wild shrimp, peeled

Add water and red onion to a frying pan, cook on high heat for 1-2 minutes. Add broccoli stems and carrot, cook for 1-2 minutes. Add broccoli and shrimp, cover and steam for 2-3 minutes. Mix ingredients for **Pungent Plum Sauce** and add to the pan. Cover and cook on low heat for 2-3 minutes. Serves four.

Pungent Plum Sauce

3 garlic cloves, peeled and
    minced

½ cup water

1/3 cup toasted sesame oil

1 tbsp. maple syrup

3 tbsp. plum jam

2-3 tbsp. shoyu

1 tsp. hot pepper flakes

½ tbsp. kuzu root starch (+2-3
    tbsp. water to dilute)

Put all ingredients, except kuzu, into a small sauce pot and cook on medium heat for 2-3 minutes. Dilute kuzu in a small amount of water and add slowly to the pot. Sauce will begin to thicken. Cook for 3-5 minutes or until kuzu becomes clear.

White Fish And Winter Veggie Stew

½ pound scrod or other white
fish

1 potato, diced

1 onion, peeled and diced

1 rutabaga, diced

2 turnips, diced

½ celery root, peeled and diced

1 carrot, diced

1 tsp. sea salt

Black pepper to taste

6 cups water

Parsley, minced

Nori strips

Bring all ingredients to a boil. Cover and cook on medium heat for 15 minutes. Add parsley and cook for 2-3 minutes. Adjust seasoning if needed. Garnish with thin strips of nori. Serves four.

Creamy Cod Chowder

2 tbsp. olive oil or butter

2 tbsp. whole grain pastry flour
(or other flour)

6 cups water

1 onion, peeled and minced

1 carrot, diced

2 celery stalks, diced

8 ounces cod, cut into small
chunks

2 bay leaves

1½ tsp. dried basil

1-2 tsp. sea salt

3 scallions, minced

Sauté flour in oil or butter. Slowly add water, stirring constantly. Add all ingredients except scallions, cover and cook on medium/low flame for 10-15 minutes. Remove ½ the soup ingredients and puree in a food processor. Return to soup. Garnish with scallions. Serves four.

Teriyaki Salmon

2 inches ginger, peeled and
  minced
2 garlic cloves, peeled and
  minced
¼ cup shoyu or tamari

½ cup water
2 tbsp. maple syrup or honey
½ pound wild salmon
1 bag mesclun greens
3-4 scallions, minced

Clean salmon and place in a frying pan. Mix ginger, garlic, shoyu, water, and maple syrup. Pour liquid ingredients over salmon and bring to a boil. Cover and reduce flame to medium. Cook for 7-10 minutes. Remove salmon from the pan and place on top of the mesclun greens. Continue cooking the liquid in the pan until reduced to 3-4 tbsp. Drizzle reduced teriyaki sauce over the salmon and mesclun greens. Garnish with scallions. Serves two.

Roasted Halibut & Miso Ginger Sauce

12 ounces halibut
¼ cup water
Juice of 1 lemon
2 tbsp. ginger juice

3 tbsp. shoyu
2 heaping tbsp. sweet white
  miso
Scallions, minced

Preheat oven to 375°. Place halibut in a baking pan with a small amount of water. Mix lemon, ginger juice (finely grate ginger and squeeze pulp), shoyu and miso until smooth and creamy. Spread mixture on top of fish. Roast for 15-20 minutes. Garnish with scallions. Serves three.

Salmon Croquettes With Dill Sauce

8-10 ounces wild salmon, diced

3 scallions, minced

½ cup whole grain bread
   crumbs

2 egg whites

2 tbsp. parsley

Sea salt & Black Pepper (to
   taste)

1 tbsp. olive oil

½ cup yogurt

1 tbsp. fresh dill

1 tbsp. lemon juice

1 tsp. prepared stoneground
   mustard

Mix diced salmon, scallions, breadcrumbs, egg whites, parsley, sea salt and pepper in a bowl or food processor (if using a food processor, pulse the ingredients but do not puree). Form into patties and fry on medium heat until lightly crisp and browned – about 3-5 minutes on each side. Combine yogurt, mustard, dill and lemon juice. Put a dollop of dill sauce on top of each croquette. Makes four croquettes.

Tasty Tuna Burgers

8-10 ounces fresh tuna, diced

6 pieces pickled ginger, minced

  1 egg, beaten

1 bunch of scallions, minced

2 tbsp. whole grain flour

1 tbsp. sesame oil

1 tbsp. powdered wasabi
  mustard

¼ cup of water

1 tbsp. shoyu

1 tbsp. honey

2 tbsp. homemade mayonnaise
  (see below)

Whole grain burger buns

Lettuce leaves

Red onion slices

Combine tuna, pickled ginger (can buy in any health food store or Asian market), egg, scallions and flour, and form into 1 inch thick patties. Fry in sesame oil until lightly browned on both sides (3-4 minutes). Place tuna burger inside a toasted whole grain bun with lettuce and freshly sliced onions. Mix wasabi powder, shoyu, homemade mayonnaise, honey, water, and pickled ginger juice. Put a dollop on top of tuna burgers. Makes four burgers.

Homemade Mayonnaise

1 whole egg + 1 egg white

1 tsp. prepared Dijon mustard

1 tbsp. apple cider vinegar

Generous pinch of sea salt

¾ cup olive oil or other oil

Puree all ingredients in the food processor, except olive oil. Slowly add olive oil in small amounts while the food processor is on – be patient this takes time. Add more sea salt if desired. You could also add fresh herbs like parsley, or chives to make an herbed mayonnaise.

Simple Shrimp & Soba

1 package soba noodles

¼ cup water

1 red onion, peeled and sliced
   into crescents

2-3 carrots, cut on thin
   diagonals

½ bunch asparagus, cut into 2
   inch pieces (trim off woody
   asparagus bottoms)

½ pound shrimp, peeled

1 red bell pepper, deseeded and
   diced

1 tbsp. hot pepper sesame oil

1 tsp. hot red pepper flakes

1 tbsp. maple syrup

3 tbsp. shoyu

Pinch cayenne pepper

2 scallions, minced

Bring water to a boil. Add noodles and cook according to instructions on the package (about 7-10 minutes). In a separate pan, water sauté onion for 1-2 minutes. Add carrots and cook 2-3 minutes. Chop off woody asparagus bottoms and discard. Cut remaining asparagus into two inch pieces and add to the pan. Add shrimp and red pepper. Cover and cook for 2 minutes. Mix hot sesame oil, hot pepper flakes, maple syrup, shoyu, cayenne pepper and ¼ cup of water, and add to the pan. Cook for 3-5 minutes. Drain cooked soba noodles. Mix shrimp and vegetables with noodles, garnish with scallions. Serves four.

BARNYARD BISTRO

Old Fashioned Chicken Soup

Vegetable Omelet

Roasted Zucchini and Chicken Sausage

Stuffed Delicata Squash with Turkey

Peanutty Fried Rice

Cobb Salad with Dulse Dressing

Sauteed Spaghetti Squash & Sausage

Jumpin Jambalya

Duck Amok in Peanut Noodles

Beef with Broccoli & Garlic Sauce

Lamb Stew

Curried Chicken Salad

Chicken &Baby Spinach Salad with Raspberry Vinaigrette

Black Beans and Bacon

Wild Rice Pilaf with Chicken & Apple Sausage Topped with
Savory Mushroom Gravy

Lazy Lamb Chops and Collard Greens

Many of the recipes in this section contain foods from all other categories too; soups, salads, grains, beans, fish, etc. It shows the many ways we could use animal products without making them the main centerpiece, but incorporating them wisely into a fully balanced meal. This way of eating reflects a traditional healthy consumption of animal products for many temperate climates, most notably the Asian and Mediterranean.

At one time in my life I was a strict vegetarian. Abstaining from meats and other animal products helped me feel better initially, but in the long term contributed to deficiencies. When I reintroduced animal foods into my diet, I did so in a healthier, more traditional way; combining them with other foods to maintain balance.

It's up to you to figure out what works best, and what your body *needs*. One client had this to say, "In my heart, I wish I was a vegetarian, but my body seems to need beef, poultry and fish to be healthy. The best comment Andrea ever gave me about eating meat was to bless the beef first before eating it: thank God and thank the cow." - Nicole Borgenicht.

When purchasing animal meat and other products, always choose the best quality; naturally raised, hormone free, antibiotic free, pastured and free range – and don't forget to bless the animal for its life. Something like, "thank you for this animal's amazing energy... now, please pass the Beef with Broccoli and Garlic Sauce."

Old Fashioned Chicken Soup

6 cups water

2 bay leaves

1 onion, peeled and diced

½ celeriac root, diced

1 red potato, diced

2 carrots, diced

3-4 organic, free-range chicken
pieces (drumsticks, wings,
etc.)

1½ tsp. sea salt

Black pepper

1 tsp. thyme

¼ cup parsley, minced

2 garlic cloves, peeled and
minced

½ cup whole grain alphabet
pasta or small pasta

Bring water, onion, celeriac root (you could substitute 2 celery stalks, diced), red potato, carrot, chicken pieces (with skin), sea salt, one shake of black pepper, and thyme to a boil. Reduce flame, cover and simmer for 35 minutes. Remove chicken pieces from liquid and cool. While chicken is cooling, add parsley, garlic and dried pasta, and continue cooking for 8-10 minutes. Discard chicken skin. Separate chicken meat from bones (dice or shred meat) and toss back into the soup. Serves six.

Sauteed Vegetable Omelet

2 tbsp. butter

½ leek, cleaned and sliced thin

3-4 cremini mushrooms, sliced
   thin

4-5 spinach leaves, finely
   chopped

4 organic eggs, beaten

2 tbsp. grated raw milk
   cheddar or swiss cheese

Sea salt

Black Pepper

In one tbsp. butter, sauté leek, mushroom and spinach on medium/high heat until soft and wilted (3-5 minutes). Remove vegetables from skillet and set aside on a plate. Add remaining butter to the pan and cook the beaten eggs on medium/low heat. Roll the pan around allowing egg to distribute evenly on the inside of the skillet. When the egg is almost fully cooked (2-3 minutes), put the cooked vegetables, grated cheese and sea salt and pepper on top of the eggs. Gently lift one side of the omelet with a spatula and fold over the vegetables and cheese. Cook an additional minute and then gently slide the omelet out of the pan and onto a plate. Serves two.

Roasted Zucchini And Chicken Sausage

2 yellow zucchini, halved and
   deseeded

2 cups Italian Rice Salad (see
   index)

2 links organic chicken sausage
   (sweet Italian style), diced

I enjoy the many varieties of naturally made sausages that are on the market today (which you'll see in the recipes that follow). If you don't like chicken sausage, substitute turkey or pork, or you could use 8 ounces of cooked chicken breast, diced. Preheat oven to 350º. Lightly oil a baking pan. Place zucchini halves into the pan, skin side down and bake, uncovered for 15 minutes or until soft. Remove from oven. In a bowl, combine Italian Rice Salad with diced chicken sausage. Place ½ cup of mixture onto each zucchini half. Put back in the oven and bake an additional 10 minutes. Serves four.

Stuffed Delicata Squash &
Turkey

2 delicata squash, deseeded and
  quartered

1 tbsp. olive oil

1 garlic clove, peeled and
  minced

1 onion, peeled and diced

2-3 celery sticks, diced

½ cup quinoa

1 cup water, vegetable or
  chicken stock

2-3 tsp. herbed sea salt

¼ cup raisins

8 ounces organic roasted
  turkey (can use dark or white
  meat), diced

2 tbsp. fresh sage, minced or 1
  tsp. dried sage

Preheat oven to 375°. Lightly oil a baking pan. Cut squash in half
lengthwise to remove seeds. Then cut each half in half to get quarters.
Place squash in baking pan and cover with aluminum foil. Bake 40
minutes or until squash is soft. While squash is cooking add olive oil to a
frying pan and sauté garlic and onion for 2-3 minutes. Add celery and
cook for 3-5 minutes or until vegetables are soft and wilted. Add quinoa,
water, raisins, diced turkey and seasonings. Bring to a boil. Cover, lower
flame and cook on simmer for 12-15 minutes. Spoon quinoa and turkey
mixture into baked squash and serve. Serves six.

Peanutty Fried Rice

2 tbsp. peanut oil

1 onion, peeled and diced

2 garlic cloves, peeled and
   minced

3-4 mushrooms, sliced thin

1 stalk broccoli, florets

¼ pound small shrimp, peeled

½ cup fresh green peas (can use
   frozen)

½ tsp. sea salt

2 eggs, beaten

8 ounces naturally cured ham,
   diced

2 cups cooked brown rice

1 tbsp. toasted sesame oil

2-3 tbsp. shoyu

1 tbsp. mirin

¼ cup water

2 scallions, minced

2 tbsp. dry roasted peanuts

In one tbsp. peanut oil, sauté onion and garlic for 2 minutes. Add mushrooms, broccoli, shrimp and green peas for 3-4 minutes. Remove vegetables from the pan and place on a plate. Add remaining tbsp. peanut oil to the pan and scramble the eggs. With a fork, break up the scrambled eggs into small pieces. Add the diced ham, cooked vegetables, and cooked rice into the pan on top of the eggs. Mix sesame oil, shoyu, mirin and water, pour into the pan. Toss all ingredients in the pan and cook 3-5 minutes. Garnish with scallions and roasted peanuts. Serves four.

Cobb Salad With Dulse Dressing

1 package mesclun greens

1 bunch baby spinach

1 red onion, peeled and sliced
   thin

2 hard boiled eggs, quartered

3-4 ounces roasted turkey
   breast, diced

4-5 black olives, pitted

2 slices naturally cured bacon,
   cook until crispy

2 tbsp. ginger juice (grate fresh
   ginger and squeeze pulp with
   hand or in a cheese cloth)

1-2 tbsp. dulse flakes

2 tbsp. brown rice syrup

1/3 cup rice vinegar

½ cup sesame oil

1/3 cup shoyu

Put mesclun greens and baby spinach in a large bowl. Attractively arrange
the onion, egg, chopped olives, and diced turkey on top of salad greens.
Whisk ginger juice, dulse flakes, rice syrup, rice vinegar, sesame oil and
shoyu. Top Cobb salad with dressing and garnish with finely chopped
crispy bacon. Serves two.

Sauteed Spaghetti Squash & Sausage

1 spaghetti squash, whole

1 tbsp. olive oil

1 onion, peeled and cut into ¼ inch crescents

3 garlic cloves, peeled and minced

1 leek, cut cleaned and cut on thin diagonals

½ hot pepper (red or green habanero or jalapeno) deseeded and diced

2 celery stalks, diced

1 cup cooked cannellini beans (can use canned beans)

1 tsp. sea salt

1 tbsp. tomato paste mixed with ½ cup water

3-4 swiss chard leaves, ripped into bite sized pieces

2 links pre-cooked organic pork sausage, cut into ¼ inch rounds (can substitute turkey or chicken sausage)

2 tbsp. fresh basil, minced

1 tbsp. fresh oregano, minced

1 tbsp. butter

Black pepper

Put spaghetti squash into a large pot with 3-4 inches of water at the bottom. Cover and cook on a high heat for 40-45 minutes or until the skin can easily be pierced. Let the squash cool. Cut squash lengthwise, and scoop out the seeds. Drag a fork through the interior of the squash to create spaghetti strands. Set aside squash strands. In a large frying pan sauté onion, garlic, leek, celery, hot pepper and sea salt. Add diluted tomato paste, swiss chard, cooked pork sausage pieces, cooked cannellini beans, basil and oregano. Cover and cook on medium heat for 5-7 minutes. Add steamed spaghetti squash and butter to the pan and cook for 2-3 minutes. Serves four.

178

Jumpin' Jambalaya

1 onion, peeled and diced

3 garlic cloves, peeled and minced

1 carrot, diced

4 links andouille or smoked turkey sausage, diced

1 cup small shrimp, peeled

2 cups canned crushed tomatoes

½ cup water

2 cups leftover or pre-cooked rice

2-3 tsp. Tabasco or other hot sauce (adjust amount to however hot you like it)

Sea salt and black pepper to taste

¼ cup parsley, minced

In a large pot combine onion, garlic, carrot, turkey sausage, shrimp, crushed tomatoes and water. Bring to a high heat, cover and cook on medium for 5 minutes. Add cooked rice, Tabasco or other hot sauce, parsley, sea salt and black pepper, and continue cooking for 3-5 minutes. Serves six people.

Duck Amok In Peanut Noodles

¼ duck (breast and wing or
   thigh and leg)

Sea salt

1 package Udon Noodles

½ cup creamy peanut butter

1/3 cup rice vinegar

1/3 cup shoyu

¼ cup maple syrup

1 garlic clove, peeled and
   minced

2 inches fresh ginger, peeled
   and diced

1 tbsp. toasted sesame oil

½ tbsp. ground szechuan
   peppercorns or hot red
   pepper flakes

¼-½ cup water for consistency

¼ cup cilantro, minced

Preheat oven to 375°. Lightly salt the duck and place in a baking pan, skin side up, and roast for 35-40 minutes. While duck is roasting, cook udon noodles according to instructions on the package. In a food processor puree peanut butter, rice vinegar, shoyu, maple syrup, garlic, ginger, hot pepper flakes and a small amount of water to achieve desired consistency. Remove duck from the oven and let cool. Discard duck skin (or eat it – don't be afraid of a little fat… it's delicious!). Pull duck apart with your fingers to get thin strips of meat. In a bowl, mix duck with drained udon noodles, and combine with peanut sauce. Garnish with cilantro. Serves six.

Beef With Broccoli &
Ginger Garlic Sauce

½ pound beef steak, sliced into quarter inch thin strips

1 tbsp. sesame oil

1 onion, peeled and cut into thin half moons

1 red pepper, deseeded and diced

2 broccoli stalks, florets and stems

3 scallions, minced (use both white and green parts)

2 cups cooked brown rice

Saute beef on medium heat for 1-2 minutes on each side. Remove beef from pan and set aside on a plate. Add onion, red pepper and broccoli to the pan and saute for 3-4 minutes or until broccoli turns bright green. Add beef back to pan with **Garlic Sauce**, cover and cook on medium for 2-3 minutes. Put ½ cup cooked brown rice on each plate, and beef with garlic sauce on top of rice. Garnish with scallions. Serves four.

Ginger Garlic Sauce

2-3 peeled garlic cloves, minced

1 inch peeled ginger, minced

½ cup water

1 tbsp. toasted sesame oil

2 tbsp. maple syrup

3 tbsp. shoyu

½ tbsp. kuzu root starch + 2-3 tbsp. water to dilute

Put all ingredients except kuzu into a small sauce pan. Cook on medium/high heat for 2-3 minutes. Dilute kuzu (or other root starch) in a small amount of water and add to the sauce pan. Cook until sauce thickens slightly.

Lamb Stew

1 lamb neck

6 cups water

1 onion, cut into chunks

2 garlic cloves, peeled and
  minced

2 small potatoes, diced

2-3 carrots, cut into 1 inch
  rounds

2 tsp. dried rosemary

1 tsp. sea salt

2-3 collard greens, diced

Bring all ingredients, except collard greens to a boil. Reduce flame to simmer, cover and cook for 25-30 minutes. Add collard greens and continue cooking for 8-10 minutes. Serves four.

Curried Chicken Salad

1 pound cooked chicken breast,
  diced

3 celery stalks, diced

2 scallions, minced (use both
  white and green parts)

3 tbsp. parsley, minced

3-4 tbsp. Homemade
  Mayonnaise (see index)

1½ tsp. curry powder

¼ tsp. sea salt

1 shake black pepper

In a large bowl combine all ingredients. Serves four.

Chicken & Baby Spinach Salad
With Raspberry Vinaigrette

8 ounces chicken breast

1 tbsp. olive oil

Sea salt

Paprika

1 bag or 4 cups baby spinach
   or mesclun greens

¼ cup cranberries

½ cup roasted walnuts

1 cup chickpeas, cooked

½ red onion, sliced into thin
   crescents

Raspberry Vinaigrette

Lightly season chicken breast with salt and paprika. On a medium heat, pan fry chicken in olive oil in for 4 minutes on each side. Remove from the pan and let cool until you can handle it without burning your fingers! Dice into 1 inch cubes. In a bowl combine diced chicken, baby spinach, cranberries, walnuts, chickpeas and red onion. Drizzle with **Raspberry Vinaigrette** just before serving. Serves two.

Spiced Raspberry Vinaigrette

2 heaping tbsp. raspberry jam

1 tbsp. Dijon mustard

¼ cup olive oil

4 tbsp. apple cider vinegar

Whisk all ingredients together.

Black Beans And Bacon

3-4 strips natural wood smoked
organic bacon (no nitrates)

1 cup black beans, soaked
overnight

2½ cups water

2 inches dried wakame (sea
vegetable)

1 medium onion, peeled and
diced

2 garlic cloves, peeled and
minced

½ tsp. thyme

1 tsp. sea salt

¼ cup parsley, minced

On a medium heat, fry bacon until crispy and remove from the pot. In the
bacon fat (yes, in the bacon fat!), sauté onion and garlic for 2-3 minutes.
Discard beans soaking water. Add beans, water and wakame to pot with
the fried onion and garlic. Bring to a boil, cover and reduce flame to
simmer for one hour and fifteen minutes. Add thyme, sea salt and parsley.
Cook for an additional 20-30 minutes. Dice crispy bacon and add to the
pot just before serving or use as a garnish. Serves six.

Wild Rice Pilaf With Sausage
& Savory Mushroom Gravy

1 cup mixed wild rice blend

2 cups water

1 tbsp. olive oil

1 onion, peeled and diced

2 celery stalk, diced

1 green apple, cored and diced

2 links smoked chicken and apple sausage (or other sausage), diced

2 tbsp. parsley, minced

½ tsp. Sea Salt

Rinse rice. Bring rice and water to a boil. Add a pinch of sea salt, lower flame, cover and simmer for 40-45 minutes. In a separate pan, sauté onion in olive oil for 2 minutes on a medium heat. Add celery, diced green apple, chicken sausage, sea salt and parsley and cook for 5-7 minutes. Combine cooked wild rice with sautéed vegetables and sausage. Top with **Savory Mushroom Gravy**. Serves four.

Savory Mushroom Gravy

6-8 mushrooms (cremini, button or other), minced

1 tbsp. butter

2 shallots, peeled and minced

1 tsp. dried thyme

1½ cups chicken stock

½ tsp. sea salt

1 tbsp. kuzu + 3 tbsp. water

Saute shallots and mushrooms for 2-3 minutes. Add thyme, chicken stock and sea salt, bring to a boil, lower flame to medium and cook 3-5 minutes. Dilute kuzu in small amount of water and add to the pot. Cook until sauce slightly thickens, about 3-4 minutes.

Lazy Lamb Chops & Collard Greens

1 tsp. olive oil

½ pound lamb chops

½ tsp. dried rosemary

Sea salt

Black pepper

4-5 collard greens, sliced thin

¼ cup water

Heat a skillet and add 1 tsp. olive oil. Season lamb chops with a sprinkling of sea salt, black pepper, and dried rosemary. Place lamb chops in the skillet and turn heat to low. Cook 6-7 minutes on each side. While lamb chops are cooking, bring water to a boil in a separate pot and throw in collard greens. Blanch on high heat for 3-4 minutes. Remove from the water, drain, and set aside. Remove cooked lamb chops from the pan. Add 1-2 tbsp. water to the lamb chop pan and toss in blanched collard greens to coat with lamb chop juice. Nestle lamb chops on top of cooked collards. Serves two.

DELICIOUS DESSERTS

Oatmeal Walnut & Raisin Cookies

Pumpkin Pudding

Chocolate Almond Mousse

Banana Ice Cream

Simple Strawberry Sorbet

Lickety Lemon Sorbet

Mixed Berry Sorbet

Blackberry Orange Sorbet

Brown Rice Crispy Treats

Berry Kanten

Puffed Amaranth and Millet Bars

Brown Rice Pudding

Coconut Almond Pudding

Chocolate Peanut Butter Truffles

Awesome Almond Brittle

Autumn Apple Crisp

Sensational Cranberry Pie

Coconut Almond Macaroons

Perfectly Poached Pears

Very Berry Whip

"Healthy" desserts can be just as delicious, if not more so, than decadent ones. We're using natural sweeteners and organic ingredients to change the quality of these desserts and make them *better*. But, even though they're considered healthier, they are still desserts and shouldn't comprise the majority of your plate – unless you have PMS, a broken heart, or were recently fired from your job.

When eating desserts, always go for the full fat and sweetened versions. If you eat no-fat, low-fat, sugar-free (artificially sweetened) desserts, your body will still crave the fat and sugar and look for it elsewhere… like in a jar of peanut butter or an insatiable sweet tooth. Let yourself have what you want, but make sure it's the best quality possible, and in moderation. Chew it well and enjoy it thoroughly.

Of course, love is the best dessert of all. Find a way to fill up your heart with love and your sweet tooth may ache less. I believe there's nothing more satisfying in this life than love …although a Chocolate Almond Mousse comes pretty darn close!

Oatmeal Walnut & Raisin Cookies

¼ cup corn oil

½ cup maple syrup

2 tsp. vanilla extract

3 tbsp. sesame tahini

2 tbsp. butter, softened

1 egg, beaten

¾ cup whole grain pastry flour

1½ cups rolled oats

½ cup walnuts, chopped

¼ cup granulated cane juice or sugar

½ cup raisins

½ tsp. cinnamon

¼ tsp. Sea salt

Preheat oven to 350º. Mix wet ingredients and dry ingredients in separate bowls, and then combine the two together. Lightly oil a cookie sheet. Using a large tablespoon, drop dough onto cookie sheet and slightly press down to ½ inch high and 3-4 inches wide. Bake for 20-25 minutes or until the edges turn brown. Let cool for 10 minutes before removing them from the baking pan. Makes ten to twelve cookies – or four monster sized cookies.

Pumpkin Pudding

1 medium sized winter squash
(buttercup, kabocha or
hokaido pumpkin)

1 cup water

2 cups rice milk or other milk

3 heaping tbsp. kuzu (diluted
in ¼ cup water)

2 tsp. pumpkin pie spice

1/3 cup maple syrup

Cut squash in half and remove the seeds, then cut squash into quarters. Put water and squash in a pot and bring to a boil. Cover and cook on medium/high heat for 15 minutes or until squash is soft (save cooking water). Let squash cool, peel skin and discard. Place squash in food processor and puree (with leftover cooking water). In a pot, put 3 cups of pureed squash, rice milk, maple syrup and pumpkin pie spice. Cook on medium/high heat for 3-4 minutes. Dilute kuzu in a small amount of water and add to the pot. Turn down flame and cook for 3-4 minutes or until thick and bubbling. Refrigerate for 1 or more hours before serving. Very Important! Do *not* wash the pumpkin pudding pot. Let it cool and then grab a large spoon, scrape down the sides of the pot, and lick the spoon clean… just like when you were a kid. Serves six.

Chocolate Almond Mousse

4 tbsp. unsweetened cocoa
  powder

4 cups almond milk

1 tsp. almond extract

1 tsp. vanilla extract

½ cup maple syrup

5 tbsp. agar-agar flakes (sea
  vegetable)

1 tbsp. almond butter

2 tbsp. roasted almonds, sliced

Combine all ingredients in a pot, except almonds and almond butter. Bring to a boil and cook on medium/high heat for 7-10 minutes or until agar dissolves. Refrigerate for 2-3 hours or until firmly gelled. Put almond butter and gelled chocolate into a food processor and blend until smooth and creamy. Top with sliced roasted almonds. Serves six.

Banana Ice Cream

6-8 ripe bananas, peeled, cut
  into chunks and frozen
  overnight

½ cup of walnuts, roasted

After my tropical fruit "dis" in the Climate Control chapter, I had redeem myself to the banana farmers around the world. Here's a simple and scrumptious way to eat bananas during the hot summer months. Freeze bananas overnight or 8-10 hours. Remove bananas from the freezer and thaw 5-10 minutes. Put bananas in a food processor and puree until you achieve ice-cream consistency. Serve immediately, topped with crushed, roasted walnuts. Serves four.

Simple Strawberry Sorbet

2 packages frozen strawberries

3-4 tbsp. grape juice
   concentrate

Fresh mint leaves

Dessert doesn't get much simpler than this. Remove strawberries from freezer and thaw 5-7 minutes. Put strawberries and grape juice concentrate into a food processor and puree until smooth and creamy. Serve immediately. Garnish with mint leaves. Serves four.

Lickety Lemon Sorbet

Juice of 5 lemons

Zest of 2 lemons (grate the
   outside peel of the lemon to
   get zest)

2 cups white grape juice

½ cup granulated cane juice or
   organic sugar

Combine all ingredients. Pour juice into an ice tray and freeze 6-8 hours or until solid. Thaw 10-15 minutes. Puree lemon cubes in a food processor until smooth. Taste and add more sugar if needed. Refreeze for 2-3 hours. Serves four.

Mixed Berry Sorbet

1 package frozen strawberries   4 tbsp. grape jam

1 package frozen raspberries   2 tbsp. raspberry jam

You could use any berries in these easy sorbet recipes. You can also buy fresh berries, rinse and freeze in plastic freezer bags. Remove frozen berries from the freezer and thaw 5-10 minutes. Put all the ingredients into a food processor and puree until creamy. Serve immediately! Serves four.

Blackberry Orange Sorbet

2 packages frozen blackberries   4 tbsp. Grape juice concentrate

¼ cup orange juice + 1 tbsp.

  orange zest

The peak of blackberry season is in the late summer, early fall. You could buy fresh ripe blackberries and freeze in plastic freezer bags. Put all the ingredients in a food processor and puree until smooth and creamy. Refreeze for 1 hour. Serves four.

Brown Rice Crispy Treats

2 cups brown rice crispy cereal

½ cup pure, creamy natural
   peanut butter

2/3 cup brown rice syrup

¼ cup roasted peanuts

¼ cup non-dairy chocolate
   chips

Kids love this recipe – and adults love it too! Mix brown rice crispy cereal and peanuts in a large bowl. Heat peanut butter and rice syrup on low flame until smooth and creamy. Pour liquid ingredients over brown rice crispy cereal and peanuts and combine thoroughly. Press ingredients into a baking pan or casserole dish and sprinkle chocolate chips on top (lightly press the chips into the mixture). Let cool for ½ an hour inside the refrigerator (if you can stand to wait that long). Cut into squares. Serves one person – just kidding! Serves six to eight, depending on how big you cut the squares.

Berry Kanten (Jello)

4 cups apple cider or juice

4 tbsp. agar-agar (sea
   vegetable)

1 cup whole blueberries

1 cup strawberries, diced

Bring apple juice and agar-agar to a boil. Lower flame to medium and cook 5-7 minutes or until agar is dissolved. Pour hot liquid over berries and chill until gelled (about 1-2 hours). Serves six.

Amaranth & Millet Energy Bars

½ cup brown rice syrup

½ cup almond butter

2-3 tbsp. honey

1 cup puffed amaranth cereal

1 cup puffed millet cereal

Sea salt

2 tbsp. raisins

2 tbsp. dried cranberries

¼ cup each of pumpkin,
    sunflower and sesame seeds,
    lightly toasted

On a medium heat, combine rice syrup, honey and almond butter until thin and pourable (about 3-4 minutes). In a mixing bowl combine puffed amaranth, puffed millet, raisins, cranberries and seeds. Pour warm almond butter mixture into the bowl and mix thoroughly. Press mixture into a casserole dish. Let cool in the refrigerator 25-30 minutes. Cut into bars. Makes 6-10 bars (depending on how big you slice them).

Brown Rice Pudding

2 cups leftover long grain
    brown rice (can use short
    grain)

1 cup rice milk, almond milk or
    other milk

¼ cup of raisins

1 tsp. cinnamon

¼ cup maple syrup

1 tsp. vanilla flavoring

1 tbsp. Tahini

This is a great way to use leftover rice. Combine ingredients in a pot and heat on top of the stove for 8-10 minutes, until most of the liquid is absorbed and pudding becomes creamy. Serves four.

Creamy Coconut Almond Rice Pudding

2 cups cooked brown basmati
rice (can use long grain)

2/3 cup coconut milk

1/3 cup almond milk

3 tbsp. unsweetened shredded
dried coconut

¼ tsp. ground allspice

¼ cup maple syrup

When I was growing up I loved Almond Joy candy bars. This rice pudding combines those two flavors, and is absolutely yummy! But, don't take my word for it, try it for yourself. Combine ingredients in a pot and bring to a boil. Lower flame to medium and cook until most of the liquid is absorbed (about 8-10 minutes). Enjoy! Serves four.

Chocolate Peanut Butter Truffles

2/3 cup natural creamy peanut
butter

½ cup powdered cane sugar

1 cup non-dairy chocolate
chips or chunks

In a bowl, use your hands to mix peanut butter and sugar until fully combined. Then roll peanut butter mixture into small balls, place on a plate and put inside the refrigerator for 20-30 minutes to set. Boil water in a double boiler and turn down the heat to simmer. Add chocolate to the upper bowl and place over the bottom pot. Stir until chocolate begins to melt. Remove top bowl from the bottom pot. Be careful, the steam from the bottom pot is hot! Stir chocolate chips around until they melt completely. Dip each peanut butter ball into the chocolate, and coat evenly. Remove ball with a spoon, and set on wax paper to dry. Yeilds 16-20 truffles.

Awesome Almond Brittle

2 cups raw almonds

½ cup honey

2 tbsp. water

2 tbsp. butter

¼ tsp. allspice

¼ tsp. cardamom

½ tsp. cinnamon

¼ tsp. sea salt, finely ground

You could use any type of nut in this recipe (peanut, walnut, hazelnut, etc.), or a combination of many – choose the nuts that you enjoy the most. Preheat oven to 350°. Place almonds on a baking sheet and roast for 10-12 minutes. Let cool. In a saucepan cook honey, water, butter, allspice, cardamom and cinnamon on a high heat for 7-10 minutes until reduced to one third the original amount. Drop almonds into the sticky liquid in the pot and coat evenly. Pour almonds on a cookie sheet or in a baking pan and flatten out with a spoon. Lightly sprinkle with finely crushed sea salt and let dry (10-15 minutes or longer). Break almonds into clusters of brittle.

Autumn Apple Crisp

3 apples, washed, cored and
  diced

¼ cup raisins

¼ cup apple juice

Juice of 1 lemon

½ cup granulated maple syrup
  or maple sugar (can use
  other sugar)

¼ cup pastry flour

1/3 cup rolled oats

¼ cup walnuts

¼ tsp. ground cardamon

½ tsp. cinammon

Pinch of coriander

1/8 tsp. sea salt

3 tbsp. softened butter

Preheat oven to 350º. Lightly oil a baking pan. In a bowl, combine apples, raisins, apple juice and lemon juice and spread evenly in the baking pan. In a bowl, combine maple sugar, pastry flour, rolled oats, walnuts, cardamom, cinnamon, coriander and sea salt. With your hands, work softened butter into the dry ingredients until evenly combined and there are no large lumps, but it resembles small crumbs. Sprinkle the crumbs on top of the apples and bake uncovered for 35-40 minutes. Serves six.

Sensational Cranberry Pie

2 cups cranberries, frozen or fresh

1 cup apple juice

¼ cup maple syrup

¼ cup sugar

1 tsp. vanilla extract

¼ cup raisins

1 pre-made whole grain pie shell

½ cup whole grain pastry flour

1/3 cup granulated cane juice

½ cup pecans, finely chopped

½ tsp. cinnamon

¼ tsp. sea salt

4 cloves, ground

4 tbsp. butter, softened

Preheat oven to 375°. Cook cranberries, apple juice, maple syrup, sugar, vanilla, and raisins on a medium heat for 25-30 minutes or until all the cranberries have popped (they pop and deflate when they are cooked). Pour cooked ingredients into a pre-made pie shell. In a bowl, combine flour, granulated cane juice, pecans, cinnamon, seal salt, and ground cloves. Mix butter into the dry ingredients with your hands until it resembles a crumble consistency. Press crumbs on top of cranberry pie. Bake 30-35 minutes or until lightly browned. Serves eight.

Coconut Almond Macaroons

2 egg whites

¼ cup granulated cane juice or
  granulated maple sugar

1 tsp. vanilla extract

1 tsp. almond extract

½ cup roasted almonds, minced

1½ cup unsweetened shredded
  dried coconut

Pinch of sea salt

Yes, yes, I know… coconuts are tropical. It's certainly okay to eat food from other climates, just don't make it the majority of your diet. And, because this is a dessert, it should *not* make up the majority of your diet! Preheat oven to 325°. Line a cookie sheet or baking tray with wax paper. Beat egg whites until foamy. Add vanilla and almond extracts, granulated cane juice and salt. Combine with shredded coconut and almonds. Drop tablespoonfuls onto cookie sheet (do not flatten). Bake for 20 minutes or until golden brown. Makes 10-14 macaroons.

Perfectly Poached Pears

4 pears, cored and diced into
  small chunks

1½ cups apple juice

1 tbsp. mulling spices

Place pears, apple juice and mulling spices into a pot and cook on a medium high heat for 10 minutes. Remove pears and chill. Strain mulling spices from apple juice and continue cooking juice until it is reduced to ¼ cup liquid (or 3 tbsp.). Drizzle over pears. Serves four.

Very Berry Whip

2 cups apple juice

3 heaping tbsp. agar flakes

1½ cup berries (blueberries, strawberries)

Bring apple juice and agar flakes to a boil. Lower flame to medium and add berries. Cook 5-7 minutes. Pour into a bowl and refrigerate for 2 hours or until completely gelled. Puree in a food processor until smooth and creamy. Serves four.

GLOSSARY

ADUKI BEANS

A traditional Japanese bean - small and dark red, with a light nutty flavor. Also known as adzuki orazuki beans.

AGAR-AGAR

This seaweed is virtually tasteless and used as a gelling agent. Agar comes in flakes or bars (also called Kanten).

AMARANTH

A tiny golden grain with a higher protein content than most grains.

ANASAZI BEANS

A maroon and white bean with a naturally sweet flavor.

APPLE CIDER VINEGAR

Flavorful vinegar made from fermented apple cider.

ARAME

A dark brown, threadlike sea vegetable rich in iron, calcium and iodine.

ARROWROOT

A thickening agent that comes from a tropical plant. Its root is dried and ground into powder.

BALSAMIC VINEGAR

This vinegar is aged for years in wooden barrels – its dark red and sweet.

BARLEY

Barley, one of the oldest cultivated grains is best eaten "hulled" because its outer hull is inedible.

BARLEY MALT

A thick brown sweetener made from roasted barley.

BLACK EYED PEAS

Medium sized ivory colored beans with a distinctive black spot on its belly.

BLACK TURTLE BEANS

Black beans with a mildly sweet flavor.

BROWN BASMATI RICE

A long grain rice with a nutty aroma and chewy texture.

BROWN RICE

A variety of types: long grain, short grain, medium grain, and sweet rice.

BROWN RICE VINEGAR

This vinegar has a low acidity and mild flavor.

BUCKWHEAT

A hearty, cereal grain that is actually a fruit seed and relative of rhubarb.

BURDOCK

A long dark root with white flesh and an earthy sweet flavor.

CANNELINI BEANS

Otherwise known as white kidney bean – creamy texture.

CAPERS

Tiny pickled flower buds, salty and sour in taste.

CHICKPEAS

Round, beige colored legumes with a creamy texture.

DAIKON

Long white radish with a pungent spicy flavor.

DULSE

A reddish purple sea vegetable that is rich in potassium and iron.

GINGER

A spicy, hot root generally used in small quantities.

GRANULATED CANE JUICE

Sweetener made from sugar cane.

GREAT NORTHERN BEANS

Medium sized white beans with a mild flavor.

HERBAMARE

An herbed sea salt seasoning that you can buy in most stores.

HIJIKI

A dark colored sea vegetable that has black stringy, spaghetti like strands.

KELP

A dark green sea vegetable rich in minerals.

KIDNEY BEANS

These are deep red, full-flavored and hearty tasting beans.

KOMBU

Dark green sea vegetable.

KUZU

A thickening starch used in desserts, sauces and home remedies. Kuzu (also know as kudzu) grows wild all over the Southeastern United States.

LENTILS

Quick cooking legumes with a peppery flavor.

LIMA BEANS

Popular white beans, also know as Butter Beans, have a delicate skin and do best cooked in salted water to keep them from falling apart.

LIMA HERBED SEA SALT

An herbed sea salt seasoning.

MAPLE SUGAR

Sweetener made by boiling maple sap.

MAPLE SYRUP

Natural sweetener made from boiling down the sap from maple trees.

MILLET

Small yellow, gluten-free grain with a nutty flavor.

MIRIN

Sweet rice cooking wine.

NAVY BEANS

Small white beans traditionally used for baking (as in baked beans).

MISO

Naturally fermented paste made from soybeans. Purchase unpasteurized miso for the best health benefits.

NORI

Green or dark purple sheets of dried sea vegetable – most commonly used to make nori maki (the rolls you eat in Japanese Sushi bars).

PINTO BEANS

Nutty flavored bean with red and brown markings on its white surface.

QUINOA

Light, fluffy high protein grain with a mild flavor and quick cooking time.

RED WINE VINEGAR

Full bodied vinegar made from aged red wine.

RICE SYRUP

Thick sweet syrup made from sprouted and fermented brown rice.

SEA SALT

A natural salt, rich in minerals, obtained from evaporating sea water.

SHITAKE MUSHROOMS

Shitake mushrooms have a meaty, earthy taste and help to lower blood cholesterol and boost the immune system.

SHOYU

Salty liquid seasoning (also known as soy sauce) made from fermented soybeans and cracked wheat.

SOBA NOODLES

Traditional Japanese noodles made from buckwheat.

SUCANAT

Dehydrated cane juice used as a natural sweetener. Also known as granulated cane juice.

TAHINI

Smooth creamy paste made from hulled, crushed sesame seeds.

TAMARI

Dark, rich and more flavorful form of shoyu (soy sauce) made without wheat.

TEMPEH

A traditionally fermented soy food – rich in vegetable protein.

TOASTED SESAME OIL

Oil extracted from toasted sesame seeds.

TOFU

A high protein soy food that is rich in calcium.

UDON NOODLES

Flat, wide noodles made from whole wheat.

UMEBOSHI VINEGAR

This is not really vinegar but salt brine. It is the liquid drawn out from the fermenting of umeboshi plums. It is both salty and sour with a light, refreshing flavor.

VANILLA EXTRACT

A flavoring extracted from the essence of vanilla beans.

WAKAME

Long green thin sea vegetable, high in minerals and trace minerals.

WHITE WINE VINEGAR

Delicate flavored vinegar made from aged white wine.

ZEST

The zest is the thin outer skin of citrus fruit.

RESOURCES

ALVARADO STREET BAKERY

Phone: (707) 585-3293

www.alvaradostreetbakery.com

Whole Grain Bread Products

COLEMAN NATURAL MEATS

colemanmeats.com/home.html

800-442-8666

Organic, naturally raised meats

DIAMOND ORGANICS

800-922-2396

www.diamondorganics.com

Organic produce and meats shipped direct

EAT WELL GUIDE

www.eatwellguide.org

Directory of grass-fed, organic meat, dairy, eggs from stores, farms and restaurants.

EDEN FOODS

888-424-EDEN (3336)

www.edenfoods.com

Organic Food Products

GOLDMINE NATURAL FOODS

800-475-FOOD (3663)

goldminenaturalfood.com

Organic natural foods and other products shipped direct

KUSHI INSTITUTE STORE

413-623-6679 or toll free 800-645-8744

www.kushistore.com

Macrobiotic specialty items

LOCAL HARVEST

http://www.localharvest.org

Locate a local farmers market, food co-op, Community Supported Agriculture (CSA), organic bio-sustainable restaurants and more.

MAINE COAST SEA VEGETABLES

207-565-2907

www.seaveg.com

Certified organic sea vegetables

NEW FARM LOCATOR

www.newfarm.org/farmlocator

Search for organic farms

NIMAN RANCH

www.nimanranch.com

Toll Free 866-808-0340

Naturally raised meats

ORGANIC FOOD DIRECTORY

www.naturalfoodnet.com

Organic growers, manufacturers, suppliers, wholesalers and more

ORGANIC CONSUMERS ASSOCIATION

www.organicconsumers.org

Promotes food safety, and organic farming

SOUTH RIVER MISO

413-369-4057

www.southrivermiso.com

Organic miso products

TRADER JOES MARKET

www.traderjoes.com

Retailer of natural and organic products

WHOLE FOODS MARKET

www.wholefoodsmarket.com

Retailer of natural and organic products

WILD BY NATURE MARKET

http://www.wildnature.com

Retailer of natural and organic products

WILD OATS MARKETS

800-494-WILD

www.wildoats.com

Retailer of organic produce and products

INDEX

Printed in the United States
67409LVS00004B/74